Gastrointestinal Physiology

Eighth Edition

LEONARD R. JOHNSON, PhD

Thomas A. Gerwin Professor of Physiology
University of Tennessee Health Sciences Center
Memphis, Tennessee

ELSEVIER
MOSBY

ELSEVIER
MOSBY

1600 John F. Kennedy Blvd.
Ste 1800
Philadelphia, PA 19103-2899

GASTROINTESTINAL PHYSIOLOGY   ISBN: 978-0-323-10085-4

Copyright © 2014, 2007 by Mosby, an imprint of Elsevier Inc.

Notices

Knowledge and best practice in this field are constantly changing. As new research and experience broaden our understanding, changes in research methods, professional practices, or medical treatment may become necessary. Practitioners and researchers must always rely on their own experience and knowledge in evaluating and using any information, methods, compounds, or experiments described herein. In using such information or methods they should be mindful of their own safety and the safety of others, including parties for whom they have a professional responsibility. With respect to any drug or pharmaceutical products identified, readers are advised to check the most current information provided (i) on procedures featured or (ii) by the manufacturer of each product to be administered, to verify the recommended dose or formula, the method and duration of administration, and contraindications. It is the responsibility of practitioners, relying on their own experience and knowledge of their patients, to make diagnoses, to determine dosages and the best treatment for each individual patient, and to take all appropriate safety precautions. To the fullest extent of the law, neither the Publisher nor the authors, contributors, or editors, assume any liability for any injury and/or damage to persons or property as a matter of products liability, negligence or otherwise, or from any use or operation of any methods, products, instructions, or ideas contained in the material herein.

Library of Congress Cataloging-in-Publication Data

Johnson, Leonard R., 1942- author.
  Gastrointestinal physiology / Leonard R. Johnson. —Eighth edition.
    p. ; cm. —(Mosby physiology monograph series)
  Preceded by Gastrointestinal physiology / edited by Leonard R. Johnson. 7th ed. c2007.
  Includes bibliographical references and index.
  ISBN 978-0-323-10085-4 (pbk.)
  I. Title. II. Series: Mosby physiology monograph series.
  [DNLM: 1. Digestive System Physiological Phenomena. WI 102]
  QP145
  612.3—dc23   2013016769

Senior Content Strategist: Elyse O'Grady
Senior Content Development Specialist: Marybeth Thiel
Content Development Specialist: Maria Holman
Publishing Services Manager: Hemamalini Rajendrababu
Project Manager: Saravanan Thavamani
Design Manager: Steven Stave
Illustrations Manager: Karen Giacomucci
Marketing Manager: Katie Alexo

Printed in China

Last digit is the print number: 9 8 7 6 5 4 3 2 1

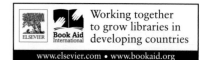

PREFACE

The first edition of *Gastrointestinal Physiology* appeared in 1977. It developed as a result of the authors' teaching experiences and the need for a book on gastrointestinal physiology written and designed for medical students and beginning graduate students. This eighth edition is directed to the same audience. As with any new edition, I believe that it is significantly better than the previous one. All chapters contain considerable amounts of new material and have been brought up-to-date with current information, without introducing undue amounts of controversy to confuse students. New figures have been added, others updated, and some chapters significantly rewritten.

Major changes in this edition are the addition of a list of "Objectives" at the beginning of chapters and "Clinical Applications" boxes within chapters. Hopefully the learning objectives will provide a guide to the important concepts and be an aid to understanding them. The material presented as clinical applications is meant to emphasize the significance of some of the basic science, provide some perspective, and increase student interest.

I am grateful to my own students for pointing out ways to improve the book. Numerous colleagues in other medical schools and professional institutions have added their suggestions and criticisms as well.

I am thankful for their interest and help, and I hope that anyone having criticisms of this edition or suggestions for improving future editions will transmit them to me.

This is the first edition appearing under sole authorship. In all previous editions, the motility chapters were written by Dr. Norman W. Weisbrodt, who has since retired. I am grateful to him for allowing me to use his material as I saw fit.

I would like to thank H.J. Ehrlein and Michael Schemann for generously allowing us to link the videos referenced in Chapters 4 and 5, which appear on the website of the Technische Universität München (http://www.wzw.tum.de/humanbiology/data/motility/34/?alt=english). The videofluoroscopy on gastrointestinal motility of dogs, pigs, and sheep was performed during the scientific studies of H.J. Ehrlein and his colleagues over a period of 25 years. This video project was supported by an educational grant from Janssen Research Foundation.

Finally, I thank Ms. Marybeth Thiel of Elsevier for suggestions and for helping with the communications and organizational work that are a necessary part of such a project.

LEONARD R. JOHNSON

CONTENTS

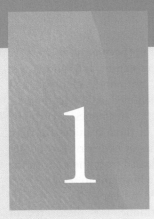

1

REGULATION: PEPTIDES OF THE GASTROINTESTINAL TRACT

OBJECTIVES

- Describe the four major functions of the gastrointestinal (GI) tract.
- Understand the differences between and significance of endocrine, paracrine, and neurocrine agents.
- Identify the major GI hormones, their functions, sites of release, and stimuli for release.
- Identify the important neurocrines and their functions in the GI tract.
- Identify the important paracrines and their functions in the GI tract.
- Understand the causes and resulting physiology of gastrinoma (Zollinger-Ellison syndrome) and pancreatic cholera (Werner Morrison syndrome).

The functions of the gastrointestinal (GI) tract are regulated by peptides, derivatives of amino acids, and a variety of mediators released from nerves. All GI hormones are peptides, but it is important to realize that not all peptides found in digestive tract mucosa are hormones. The GI tract peptides can be divided into endocrines, paracrines, and neurocrines, depending on the method by which the peptide is delivered to its target site.

Endocrines, or **hormones,** are released into the general circulation and reach all tissues (unless these substances are excluded from the brain by the blood-brain barrier). Specificity is a property of the target tissue itself. Specific receptors, which recognize and bind the hormone, are present on its target tissues and absent from others. There are five established GI hormones; in addition, some GI peptides are released from endocrine cells into the blood but have no known physiologic function. Conversely, several peptides have been isolated from mucosal tissue and have potent GI effects, but no mechanism for their physiologic release has been found. Members of these latter two groups are classified as candidate hormones.

Paracrines are released from endocrine cells and diffuse through the extracellular space to their target tissues. Their effects are limited by the short distances necessary for diffusion. Nevertheless, these agents can affect large areas of the digestive tract by virtue of the scattered and abundant distributions of the cells containing them. A paracrine agent can also act on endocrine cells. Thus a paracrine may release or inhibit the release of an endocrine substance, thereby ultimately regulating a process remote from its origin. Histamine, a derivative of the amino acid histidine, is an important regulatory agent that acts as a paracrine.

Some GI peptides are located in nerves and may act as **neurocrines** or neurotransmitters. A neurocrine is released near its target tissue and needs only to diffuse across a short synaptic gap. Neurocrines conceivably may stimulate or inhibit the release of endocrines or paracrines. **Acetylcholine** (ACh), although not a peptide, is an important neuroregulator in the GI tract. One of its actions is to stimulate acid secretion from the gastric parietal cells.

GENERAL CHARACTERISTICS

The GI tract is the largest endocrine organ in the body, and its hormones were the first to be discovered. The word *hormone* was coined by W. B. Hardy and used by Starling in 1905 to describe secretin and gastrin and to convey the concept of bloodborne chemical messengers. The GI hormones are released from the mucosa of the stomach and small intestine by nervous activity, distention, and chemical stimulation coincident with the intake of food. Released into the portal circulation, the GI hormones pass through the liver to the heart and back to the digestive system to regulate its movements, secretions, and growth. These hormones also regulate the growth of the mucosa of the stomach and small and large intestines, as well as the growth of the exocrine pancreas.

The GI peptides have many different types of actions. Their effects on water, electrolyte, and enzyme secretion are well known, but they also influence motility, growth, and release of other hormones, as well as intestinal absorption. Many of these actions overlap; two or more GI peptides may affect the same process in the same direction, or they may inhibit each other. Many of the demonstrated actions of these peptides are pharmacologic and do not occur under normal circumstances. This chapter is concerned primarily with the physiologic effects of the GI peptides.

The actions of the GI peptides also may vary in both degree and direction among species. The actions discussed in the remainder of this chapter are those occurring in humans.

DISCOVERY

Four steps are required to establish the existence of a GI hormone. First, a physiologic event such as a meal must be demonstrated to provide the stimulus to one part of the digestive tract that subsequently alters the activity in another part. Second, the effect must persist after all nervous connections between the two parts of the GI tract have been severed. Third, from the site of application of the stimulus a substance must be isolated that, when injected into the blood, mimics the effect of the stimulus. Fourth, the substance must be identified chemically, and its structure must be confirmed by synthesis.

Five GI peptides have achieved full status as hormones. They are secretin, gastrin, cholecystokinin (CCK), gastric inhibitory peptide (GIP), and motilin. There is also an extensive list of "candidate" hormones whose significance has not been established. This list includes several chemically defined peptides that have significant actions in physiology or pathology but whose hormonal status has not been proved. These are pancreatic polypeptide, neurotensin, and substance P. In addition, two known hormones, glucagon and somatostatin, have been identified in GI tract mucosa; their possible function as GI hormones is currently being investigated. Some of these peptides function physiologically as paracrines or neurocrines. Another GI peptide, **Ghrelin,** is released from the body of the stomach and functions as a hormone to regulate food intake. This topic is covered in Chapter 13.

Secretin, the first hormone, was discovered in 1902 by Bayliss and Starling and was described as a substance, released from the duodenal mucosa by hydrochloric acid, that stimulated pancreatic bicarbonate and fluid secretion. Jorpes and Mutt isolated it and identified its amino acid sequence in 1966. It was synthesized by Bodanszky and coworkers later the same year.

Edkins discovered gastrin in 1905, stating to the Royal Society that "in the process of the absorption of digested food in the stomach a substance may be separated from the cells of the mucous membrane which, passing into the blood or lymph, later stimulates the secretory cells of the stomach to functional activity." For 43 years investigators were preoccupied by the controversy over the existence of gastrin. The debate intensified when Popielski demonstrated that histamine, a ubiquitous substance present in large quantities throughout the body (including the gastric mucosa), was a powerful gastric secretagogue. In 1938 Komarov demonstrated that gastrin was a polypeptide and was different from histamine. By 1964 Gregory and his colleagues had extracted and isolated hog gastrin; Kenner and his group synthesized it the same year. After 60 years all of the criteria for establishing the existence of a GI hormone had been satisfied.

In 1928 Ivy and Oldberg described a humoral mechanism for the stimulation of gallbladder contraction initiated by the presence of fat in the intestine. The hormone was named cholecystokinin after its primary action. The only controversy involving CCK was a mild one over nomenclature. In 1943 Harper and Raper described a hormone released from the small intestine that stimulated pancreatic enzyme secretion and accordingly named it *pancreozymin.* As Jorpes and Mutt carried out the purification of these two substances in 1968, it became obvious that both properties resided in the same peptide. For the sake of convenience and because it was the first action described, this hormone is called CCK.

In 1969 Brown and his coworkers described the purification of a powerful enterogastrone from intestinal mucosa. Enterogastrone literally means a substance from the intestine (entero-) that inhibits (-one) the stomach (gastr-). By 1971 this peptide had been purified, isolated, sequenced, and named gastric inhibitory peptide for its ability to inhibit gastric secretion. Released from the intestinal mucosa by fat and glucose, GIP also stimulates insulin release. Following proof that the release of insulin was a physiologic action of the peptide, GIP became the fourth GI hormone. The insulinotropic effect of GIP requires elevated amounts of serum glucose. For this reason, and because it is doubtful whether the inhibitory effects of the peptide on the stomach are physiologic, it has been suggested that its name be changed to glucose-dependent insulinotropic peptide. In either case it is still referred to as GIP.

Brown and his coworkers also described the purification of motilin in the early 1970s. Motilin is a linear 22–amino acid peptide purified from the upper small intestine. During fasting it is released cyclically and stimulates upper GI motility. Its release is under neural control and accounts for the interdigestive migrating myoelectric complex.

CHEMISTRY

The GI hormones and some related peptides can be divided into two structurally homologous families. The first consists of gastrin (Fig. 1-1) and CCK (Fig. 1-2). The five carboxyl-terminal (C-terminal) amino acids are identical in these two hormones. All the biologic activity of gastrin can be reproduced by the four C-terminal amino acids. This tetrapeptide, then, is the minimum fragment of gastrin needed for strong activity and is about one sixth as active as the whole 17–amino acid molecule. The sixth amino acid from the C-terminus of gastrin is tyrosine, which may or may not be sulfated. When sulfated, the hormone is called gastrin II. Both forms occur with equal frequency in nature. The amino-terminus (N-terminus) of gastrin is pyroglutamyl, and the C-terminus is phenylalamide (see Fig. 1-1). The NH_2 group following Phe does not signify that this is the N-terminus; rather,

it indicates that this C-terminal amino acid is amidated. These alterations in structure protect the molecules from aminopeptidases and carboxypeptidases and allow most of them to pass through the liver without being inactivated.

Gastrin is first synthesized as a large, biologically inactive precursor called progastrin. A glycine-extended (**G-Gly**) form of gastrin is then formed by endoproteolytic processing within the G cells. G-Gly is the substrate for an amidation reaction that results in the formation of the mature, amidated gastrin. The C-terminal amide moiety is required for full biologic activity mediated by gastrin/CCK-2 receptors. Receptors for CCK and gastrin were originally called the CCK-A and CCK-B receptors, respectively; the

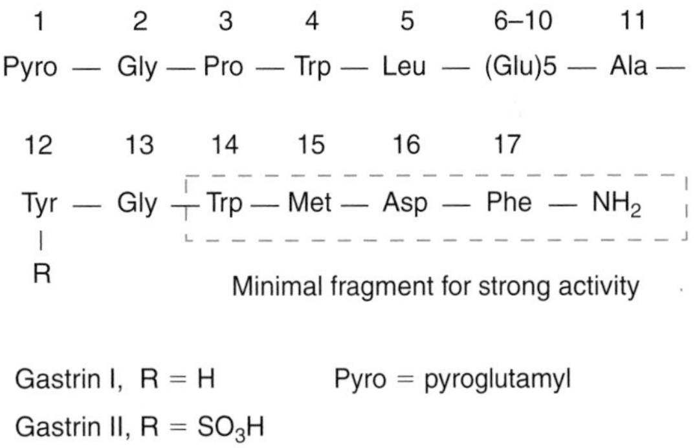

FIGURE 1-1 ■ Structure of human little gastrin (G 17).

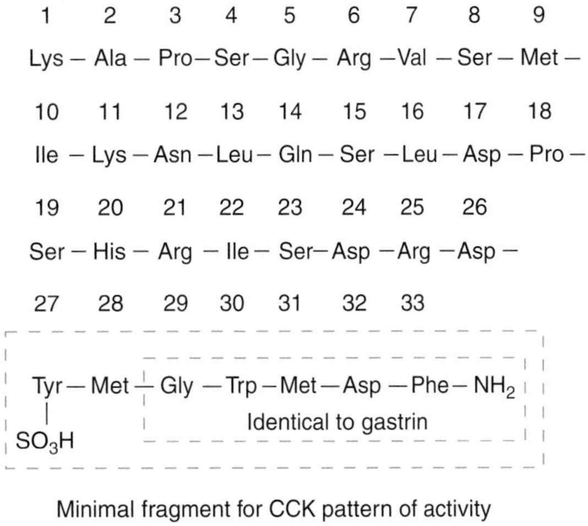

FIGURE 1-2 ■ Structure of porcine cholecystokinin (CCK).

nomenclature has been changed to CCK-1 and CCK-2. G-Gly does not stimulate the gastrin/CCK-2 receptor but instead activates its own receptor, thus leading to the activation of Jun kinase and trophic effects.

CCK, which has 33 amino acids, contains a sulfated tyrosyl residue in position 7 from the C-terminus (see Fig. 1-2). CCK can activate gastrin receptors (e.g., those for acid secretion, also called CCK-2 receptors); gastrin can activate CCK receptors (e.g., those for gallbladder contraction, also called CCK-1 receptors). Each hormone, however, is more potent at its own receptor than at those of its homologue. CCK is always sulfated in nature, and desulfation produces a peptide with the gastrin pattern of activity. The minimally active fragment for the CCK pattern of activity is therefore the C-terminal heptapeptide.

In summary, peptides belonging to the gastrin/CCK family having a tyrosyl residue in position 6 from the C-terminus or an unsulfated one in position 7 possess the gastrin pattern of activity and act on CCK-2 receptors—strong stimulation of gastric acid secretion and weak contraction of the gallbladder. Peptides with a sulfated tyrosyl residue in position 7 act on CCK-1 receptors, have cholecystokinetic potency, and are weak stimulators of gastric acid secretion. Obviously the tetrapeptide itself and all fragments less than seven amino acids long possess gastrin-like activity.

The second group of peptides is homologous to secretin and includes **vasoactive intestinal peptide** (VIP), GIP, and **glucagon,** in addition to secretin (Fig. 1-3).

Secretin has 27 amino acids, all of which are required for substantial activity. Pancreatic glucagon has 29 amino acids, 14 of which are identical to those of secretin. Glucagon-like immunoreactivity has been isolated from the small intestine, but the physiologic significance of this **enteroglucagon** has not been established. Glucagon has no active fragment, and, like secretin, the whole molecule is required before any activity is observed. Evidence indicates that secretin exists as a helix; thus the entire amino acid sequence may be necessary to form a tertiary structure with biologic activity.

GIP and VIP each have nine amino acids that are identical to those of secretin. Each has many of the same actions as those of secretin and glucagon. This group of peptides is discussed in greater detail later in the chapter.

Most peptide hormones are heterogeneous and occur in two or more molecular forms. Gastrin, secretin, and CCK all have been shown to exist in more than one form. Gastrin was originally isolated from hog antral mucosa as a heptadecapeptide (see Fig. 1-1), which is now referred to as little gastrin (G 17). It accounts for 90% of antral gastrin. Yalow and Berson demonstrated heterogeneity by showing that the major component of gastrin immunoactivity in the serum was a larger molecule that they called big gastrin. On isolation, big gastrin was found to contain 34 amino acids; hence it is called G 34. Trypsin splits G 34 to yield G 17 plus a heptadecapeptide different from G 17. Therefore, G 34 is not simply a dimer of G 17.

	*	1	2	3	4	5	6	7	8	9	10	11	12	13	14	15
Secretin	(27)	His–	Ser–	Asp–	Gly–	Thr–	Phe–	Thr–	Ser–	Glu–	Leu–	Ser–	Arg–	Leu–	Arg–	Asp–
VIP	(28)				Ala–	Val–			Asp–	Asn–	Tyr–	Thr–				Lys–
GIP	(42)	Tyr–	Ala–	Glu–				Ile–		Asp–	Tyr–		Ile–	Ala–	Met	
Glucagon	(29)			Gln–						Asp–	Tyr–		Lys–	Tyr–	Leu	

	16	17	18	19	20	21	22	23	24	25	26	27	28	29
Secretin	Ser–	Ala–	Arg–	Leu–	Gln–	Arg–	Leu–	Leu–	Gln–	Gly–	Leu–	Val–	NH_2–	
VIP	Gln–	Met–	Ala–	Val–	Lys–	Lys–	Tyr–		Asn–	Ser–	Ile–	Leu–	Asn–	NH_2–
GIP	Lys–	Ile		Gln–		Asp–	Phe–	Val–	Asn–	Trp–		Leu–	Ala–	Gln –14 more
Glucagon		Arg–		Ala–		Asp–	Phe–	Val–		Trp–		Met–	Asp–	Thr

* Total amino acid residues
  Blank spaces indicate residues identical to those in secretin.

FIGURE 1-3 ■ Structures of the secretin family of peptides. GIP, gastric inhibitory peptide; VIP, vasoactive intestinal peptide.

An additional gastrin molecule (G 14) has been isolated from tissue and contains the C-terminal tetradecapeptide of gastrin. Current evidence indicates that most G 17 is produced from pro G 17 and most G 34 is derived from pro G 34. Thus G 34 is not a necessary intermediate in the production of G 17.

During the interdigestive (basal) state, most human serum gastrin is G 34. Unlike those of other species, the duodenal mucosa of humans contains significant amounts of gastrin. This is primarily G 34 and is released in small amounts during the basal state. After a meal, a large quantity of antral gastrin, primarily G 17, is released and provides most of the stimulus for gastric acid secretion. Smaller amounts of G 34 are released from both the antral and the duodenal mucosa. G 17 and G 34 are equipotent, although the half-life of G 34 is 38 minutes and that of G 17 is approximately 7 minutes. The plasma concentration of gastrin in fasting humans is 10 to 30 pmol/L, and it doubles or triples during the response to a normal mixed meal.

DISTRIBUTION AND RELEASE

The GI hormones are located in endocrine cells scattered throughout the GI mucosa from the stomach through the colon. The cells containing individual hormones are not clumped together but are dispersed among the epithelial cells. The nature of this distribution makes it virtually impossible to remove the source of one of the GI hormones surgically and examine the effect of its absence without compromising the digestive function of the animal.

The endocrine cells of the gut are members of a widely distributed system termed **amine precursor uptake decarboxylation** (APUD) cells. These cells all are derived from neuroendocrine-programmed cells originating in the embryonic ectoblast.

The distributions of the individual GI hormones are shown in Figure 1-4. Gastrin is most abundant in the antral and duodenal mucosa. Most of its release under physiologic conditions is from the antrum. Secretin, CCK, GIP, and motilin are found in the duodenum and jejunum.

Ultrastructurally, GI endocrine cells have hormone-containing granules concentrated at their bases, close to the capillaries. The granules discharge, thereby releasing their hormones in response to events that are either the direct or the indirect result of neural, physical, and chemical stimuli associated with eating a meal and the presence of that meal within the digestive tract. These endocrine cells have microvilli on their apical borders that presumably contain receptors for sampling the luminal contents.

Table 1-1 lists the stimuli that are physiologically important releasers of the GI hormones. Gastrin and motilin are the only hormones shown to be released directly by neural stimulation. Protein in the form of peptides and single amino acids releases both gastrin and CCK. Fatty acids containing eight or more carbon atoms or their monoglycerides are the most potent stimuli for CCK release. Fat must be broken down into an absorbable form before release of CCK, thus providing evidence that the receptors for release are triggered during the process of absorption.

Evidence indicates that intestinal releasing factors secreted into the intestine of certain species, including humans, stimulate the release of CCK. Pancreatic enzymes inactivate these releasing factors. The ingestion and presence of a meal in the intestine result in

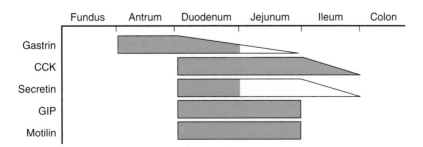

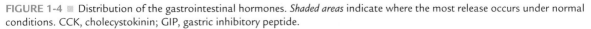

FIGURE 1-4 ■ Distribution of the gastrointestinal hormones. *Shaded areas* indicate where the most release occurs under normal conditions. CCK, cholecystokinin; GIP, gastric inhibitory peptide.

TABLE 1-1

Releasers of Gastrointestinal Hormones

	HORMONE				
Releaser	Gastrin	CCK	Secretin	GIP	Motilin
Protein	S	S	0	S	0
Fat	0	S	S-	S	S-
Carbohydrate	0	0	0	S	0
Acid	I	S-	S	0	S-
Distention	S	0	0	0	0
Nerve	S	0	0	0	S

CCK, cholecystokinin; GIP, gastric inhibitory peptide; I, inhibits release physiologically; S, physiologic stimulus for release; S-, of secondary importance; 0, no effect.

temporary binding of trypsin and other proteases and allow the releasing factors to remain active and stimulate CCK secretion. Thus this mechanism acts as a negative feedback control on pancreatic enzyme secretion.

Carbohydrate, the remaining major foodstuff, does not alter the release of gastrin, secretin, or CCK to a significant extent but does stimulate GIP release. GIP also is released by fat and protein. The strongest stimulus for secretin release is H^+. Secretin is released when the pH in the duodenum falls below 4.5. Secretin also is released by fatty acids. This may be a significant mechanism for secretin release because the concentration of fatty acids in the lumen is often high. CCK can also be released by acid, but except during hypersecretion of acid, the physiologic significance of this mechanism of release has not been established. The purely physical stimulus of distention activates antral receptors and causes gastrin release; for example, inflating a balloon in the antrum releases gastrin. During a meal the pressure of ingested food initiates this response. The magnitude of the response is not as great as originally believed, however, and the contribution of distention to the total amount of gastrin released in humans probably is minor. Gastrin also can be released by calcium, decaffeinated coffee, and wine. Pure alcohol in the same concentration as that of wine does not release gastrin but does stimulate acid secretion. Motilin is released cyclically (approximately every 90 minutes) during fasting. This release is prevented by atropine and ingestion of a mixed meal. Acid and fat in the duodenum, however, increase motilin release.

In addition to releasing secretin, acid exerts an important negative feedback control of gastrin release. Acidification of the antral mucosa below a pH of 3.5 inhibits gastrin release. Patients with atrophic gastritis, pernicious anemia, or other conditions characterized by the chronic decrease of acid-secreting cells and hyposecretion of acid may have extremely high serum concentrations of gastrin because of the absence of this inhibitory mechanism.

Hormones alter the release of GI peptides in several instances. Both secretin and glucagon, for example, inhibit gastrin release. CCK has been shown to stimulate glucagon release, and four GI hormones (secretin, gastrin, CCK, and GIP) increase insulin secretion. Elevated serum calcium stimulates both gastrin and CCK release. It is doubtful whether any of these mechanisms, with the exception of release of insulin by GIP, play a role in normal GI physiology. Some mechanisms, however, may become important when circulating levels of hormones or calcium are altered by disease.

ACTIONS AND INTERACTIONS

The effects of pure GI hormones have been tested on almost every secretory, motor, and absorptive function of the GI tract. Each peptide has some action on almost every target tested. Even though large doses of hormone sometimes are necessary to produce an effect, either stimulatory or inhibitory, these tests indicate that receptors for each hormone are present on most target tissues. The myriad activities possessed by these peptides are summarized in Table 1-2.

The important physiologic actions of the GI hormones are depicted in Table 1-3. Numerous guidelines have been proposed for determining whether an action is physiologic. The action should occur in response to endogenous hormone released by normal stimuli (i.e., those present during a meal). In other words, an exogenous dose of hormone should produce the effect in question without elevating serum hormone levels above those produced by a meal. An acceptable guideline for exogenous infusion is a dose that produces 50% of the maximal response (D_{50}) of the primary action of the hormone. The hormone should be administered as a continuous intravenous infusion rather than as a single bolus because the a bolus produces transient, unphysiologically high serum levels.

TABLE 1-2
Actions of Gastrointestinal Hormones

Action	HORMONE				
	Gastrin	CCK	Secretin	GIP	Motilin
Acid secretion	S	S	I	I	
Gastric emptying	I	I	I	I	
Pancreatic HCO_3^- secretion	S	S	S	0	
Pancreatic HCO_3^- enzyme secretion	S	S	S	0	
Bile HCO_3^- secretion	S	S	S	0	
Gallbladder contraction	S	S	S		
Gastric motility	S	S	I	I	S
Intestinal motility	S	S	I		S
Insulin release	S	S	S	S	
Mucosal growth	S	S	I		
Pancreatic growth	S	S	S		

CCK, cholecystokinin; GIP, gastric inhibitory peptide; HCO_3^-, bicarbonate; I, inhibits; S, stimulates;
0, no effect; *blank spaces,* not yet tested.

TABLE 1-3
Important Actions of Gastrointestinal Hormones

Action	HORMONE				
	Gastrin	CCK	Secretin	GIP	Motilin
Acid secretion	S		I	I	
Pancreatic HCO_3^- secretion		S	S		
Pancreatic enzyme secretion		S			
Bile HCO_3^- secretion			S		
Gallbladder contraction		S			
Gastric emptying		I			
Insulin release			S		
Mucosal growth	S				
Pancreatic growth		S	S		
Gastric motility					S
Intestinal motility					S

CCK, cholecystokinin; GIP, gastric inhibitory peptide; HCO_3^-, bicarbonate; I, inhibits; S, stimulates.

The primary action of gastrin is the stimulation of gastric acid secretion. It does this by causing the release of histamine (a potent acid secretagogue) from the **enterochromaffin-like** (ECL) cells of the stomach and by direct action on the parietal cells. Gastrin is the most important regulator of gastric acid secretion. There is considerable debate on the role of gastrin in regulating the tone of the lower esophageal sphincter, and the bulk of the evidence indicates no normal role for gastrin in regulation.

One of the most important and more recently discovered actions of GI hormones is their trophic activity. Gastrin stimulates synthesis of ribonucleic acid (RNA), protein, and deoxyribonucleic acid (DNA), as well as growth of the mucosa of the small intestine, colon, and oxyntic gland area of the stomach. If most endogenous gastrin is removed by antrectomy, these tissues atrophy. Exogenous gastrin prevents this atrophy. Patients with tumors that constantly secrete gastrin exhibit hyperplasia and hypertrophy of the acid-secreting portion of the stomach. Gastrin also stimulates the growth of ECL cells. Continued hypersecretion of gastrin results in ECL cell hyperplasia, which may develop into carcinoid tumors. The trophic effects of gastrin are restricted to GI tissues and are counteracted by secretin. The trophic action of gastrin is a direct effect that can be demonstrated in tissue culture.

As mentioned previously, G-Gly also has trophic effects. G-Gly is far less potent (by at least four orders of magnitude) than gastrin in stimulating gastric acid secretion. However, G-Gly is stored in gut tissues, is secreted with gastrin from antral G cells, and reaches concentrations in plasma equal to those of gastrin. Although antagonists of the CCK-B/gastrin receptor block the trophic effects of gastrin, they have no effect on the growth-promoting actions of G-Gly. Additional evidence suggests that the growth-related receptors for G-Gly work in concert with gastrin to regulate the functional development of the gut.

The primary effect of secretin is the stimulation of pancreatic fluid and bicarbonate secretion; one of the primary actions of CCK is the stimulation of pancreatic enzyme secretion. In addition, CCK has a physiologically important interaction in potentiating the primary effect of secretin. Thus CCK greatly increases the pancreatic bicarbonate response to low circulating levels of secretin.

Both CCK and secretin also stimulate the growth of the exocrine pancreas. CCK exerts a stronger effect than secretin, but the combination of the two hormones produces a potentiated response in rats that is truly remarkable. It is likely that the effects of these two hormones on pancreatic growth are as important as their effects on pancreatic secretion.

In addition to its effects on the pancreas, secretin stimulates biliary secretion of fluid and bicarbonate. This action is shared by CCK, but secretin is the most potent choleretic of the GI hormones. In dogs, secretin is a potent inhibitor of gastrin-stimulated acid secretion. This action is probably not physiologically important in humans. The ability of secretin to inhibit acid secretion may be important in some human diseases, however, and students should be aware of this action. Secretin has been nicknamed "nature's antacid" because almost all its actions reduce the amount of acid in the duodenum. The only known exception to this statement is secretin's pepsigogic activity. Secretin is second only to ACh in promoting pepsinogen secretion from the chief cells of the stomach. Because only small amounts of secretin are released under normal circumstances, it is doubtful whether secretin stimulates pepsin secretion physiologically.

In addition to its physiologic actions on pancreatic and biliary secretion, CCK regulates gallbladder contraction and gastric emptying. Of the GI peptides, CCK is the most potent regulator of gallbladder contraction; it is approximately 100 times more effective than the gastrin tetrapeptide in contracting the gallbladder. CCK causes significant inhibition of gastric emptying in doses equal to the D_{50} of pancreatic secretion. Gastrin also inhibits gastric emptying, but the effective dose is approximately 6 times the D_{50} for stimulation of acid secretion by gastrin. These data support the conclusions that CCK physiologically inhibits gastric emptying and gastrin does not.

CCK also functions to regulate food intake. It was the first satiety hormone to be discovered, and this action is fully covered in Chapter 13.

Several peptides, including secretin and GIP, are enterogastrones. GIP was originally discovered because of its ability to inhibit gastric acid secretion, and it may well have been the original enterogastrone described by Ivy and Farrell in 1925. Its action has not been established as physiologically significant in the innervated stomach. GIP, however, is a strong stimulator of insulin release and is responsible for the fact that an oral glucose load releases more insulin and is metabolized more rapidly than an equal amount of glucose administered intravenously.

Motilin stimulates the so-called migrating motility or myoelectric complex that moves through the stomach and small bowel every 90 minutes in the fasted GI tract. Its cyclic release into the blood is inhibited by the ingestion of a meal. This is the only known function to this peptide.

CANDIDATE HORMONES

Earlier in this chapter, certain peptides isolated from digestive tract tissue were mentioned that may, at a later date, qualify as hormones. These often are referred to as *candidate,* or *putative, hormones.* Many have been proposed, but interest is greatest for those listed in Table 1-4. Enteroglucagon belongs to the secretin family. Pancreatic polypeptide and peptide YY (tyrosine-tyrosine) belong to a separate family and are unrelated to either gastrin or secretin.

Pancreatic polypeptide was first identified as a minor impurity in insulin. It was then isolated and found to be a linear peptide with 36 amino acid residues. From a physiologic viewpoint the most important action of pancreatic polypeptide is the inhibition of both pancreatic bicarbonate and enzyme secretion because this effect has the lowest dose requirement. Most constituents of a meal release pancreatic polypeptide, and the serum levels reached are sufficient to

TABLE 1-4		
Candidate Hormones		
Peptide	*Released By*	*Action(s)*
Pancreatic polypeptide	Protein Fat Glucose	$\downarrow$Pancreatic HCO_3^- and enzyme secretion
Peptide YY	Fat	$\downarrow$Gastric secretion $\downarrow$Gastric emptying
Enteroglucagon	Hexose Fat	$\downarrow$Gastric secretion $\downarrow$Gastric emptying $\uparrow$Insulin release

$\downarrow$, inhibits; $\uparrow$, stimulates; HCO_3^-, bicarbonate.

inhibit pancreatic secretion. Because the peak rate of pancreatic secretion during a meal is less than the maximal rate that can be achieved with exogenous stimuli, it is possible that pancreatic polypeptide modulates this response under normal conditions. Before it can be concluded that pancreatic polypeptide is responsible for the physiologic inhibition of pancreatic secretion, it must be shown that this actually occurs and that pancreatic polypeptide is the causative agent. The fact that the peptide is located in the pancreas and cannot be removed without also removing its target organ makes this evidence difficult to obtain.

Peptide YY was discovered in porcine small intestine and was named for its N-terminal and C-terminal amino acid residues—both tyrosines. Of its 36 amino acid residues, 18 are identical to those of pancreatic polypeptide. Peptide YY is released by meals, especially by fat. It may appear in plasma in concentrations sufficient to inhibit gastric secretion and emptying and thus qualifies as an enterogastrone. Its effects do not appear to be direct in that it does not inhibit secretion in response to gastrin or histamine. It does inhibit neurally stimulated secretion, but its final status as an enterogastrone has not been determined. Peptide YY also inhibits intestinal motility, and this effect is believed by some investigators to enhance luminal nutrient digestion and absorption.

The enteroglucagons are products of the same gene processed in the pancreatic alpha cell to form glucagon. The intestinal L cell makes three forms of glucagon, one of which, glucagon-like peptide-1 (GLP-1), may have important physiologic actions. This 30–amino acid peptide is a potent insulin releaser, even in the absence of hyperglycemia, and it also inhibits gastric secretion and emptying. GLP-1 may mediate the so-called ileal brake—the inhibition of gastric and pancreatic secretion and motility that occurs when lipids and/or carbohydrates are infused into the ileum in amounts sufficient to cause malabsorption.

NEUROCRINES

All GI peptides were once believed to originate from endocrine cells and therefore to be either hormones or candidate hormones. With the advent of sophisticated immunocytochemical techniques for tissue localization of peptides, it became apparent that many

of these peptides were contained within the nerves of the gut.

Numerous peptides have been found in both the brain and the digestive tract mucosa. The first of these to be isolated was substance P, which in the GI tract stimulates intestinal motility and gallbladder contraction. The only other peptide isolated from both the brain and gut and known to have an identical structure in both sites is neurotensin. Neurotensin increases blood glucose by stimulating glycogenolysis and glucagon release and inhibiting insulin release. Other peptides have been isolated from one site and identified by radioimmunoassay in the other. These include motilin, CCK, and VIP, which were first isolated from the gut. Enkephalin, somatostatin, and thyrotropin-releasing factor were first isolated from the brain and later found in the gut. Gastrin, VIP, somatostatin, and enkephalin also are present in the nerves of the gut.

Three peptides have important physiologic functions in the gut as neurocrines (listed in Table 1-5). Originally investigators thought that VIP was found in gut endocrine cells, but VIP is now known to be localized within the gut exclusively within nerves. It physiologically mediates the relaxation of GI smooth muscle. Smooth muscle is innervated by VIP-containing fibers, and VIP is released during relaxation. VIP relaxes smooth muscle, and VIP antiserum blocks neurally induced relaxation. In addition, strong evidence indicates that VIP physiologically mediates relaxation of smooth muscle in blood vessels and thus may be responsible for vasodilation. Besides these effects, VIP has many of the actions of its relatives, secretin and GIP, when it is injected into the bloodstream. It stimulates pancreatic secretion, inhibits gastric secretion, and

TABLE 1-5		
Neurocrines		
Peptide	*Location*	*Action*
VIP	Mucosa and muscle of gut	Relaxation of gut smooth muscle
GRP or bombesin	Gastric mucosa	↑Gastrin release
Enkephalins	Mucosa and muscle of gut	↑Smooth muscle tone

GRP, gastrin-releasing peptide; VIP, vasoactive intestinal peptide; ↑, stimulates.

stimulates intestinal secretion. Many of the effects of VIP on smooth muscle are mediated by nitric oxide (NO); VIP stimulates the synthesis of this potent smooth muscle relaxant.

Numerous biologically active peptides have been isolated from amphibian skin and later found to have mammalian counterparts. One of these, called *bombesin* after the species of frog from which it was isolated, is a potent releaser of gastrin. The mammalian counterpart of bombesin is gastrin-releasing peptide (GRP), which has been found in the nerves of the gastric mucosa. GRP is released by vagal stimulation and mediates the vagal release of gastrin. Luminal protein digestion products may also stimulate gastrin release through a GRP-mediated mechanism.

Two pentapeptides isolated from pig and calf brains activate opiate receptors and are called *enkephalins.* They are identical except that the C-terminal amino acid is methionine in one and leucine in the other. These compounds are present in nerves within both the smooth muscle and the mucosa of the GI tract. Opiate receptors on circular smooth muscle cells mediate contraction, and leuenkephalin and metenkephalin cause contraction of the lower esophageal, pyloric, and ileocecal sphincters. The enkephalins function physiologically at these sites and also may be an intricate part of the peristaltic mechanism. The effect of opiates on intestinal motility is to slow transit of material through the gut. These peptides also inhibit intestinal secretion. The combination of these actions probably accounts for the effectiveness of opiates in treating diarrhea.

Absent from Table 1-5 is pituitary adenylate cyclase–activating peptide (PACAP), the newest member of the secretin family. If somatostatin is blocked, injection of PACAP stimulates the release of histamine from ECL cells and therefore stimulates acid secretion. PACAP also stimulates ECL cell growth, so its actions are similar to those of gastrin. It may be a significant neural mediator of ECL cell function, but direct evidence that ECL cells are innervated by PACAP-containing fibers is missing.

PARACRINES

Paracrines are like hormones in that they are released from endocrine cells. They are similar to neurocrines because they interact with receptors close to the point of their release. The biologic significance of an endocrine can be assessed by correlating physiologic events with changes in blood levels of the hormone in question. Because the area of release of both paracrines and neurocrines is restricted, no comparable methods are available for proving the biologic significance of one of these agents. Current experiments examine the effects of specific pharmacologic blockers or antisera directed toward these substances. In vitro perfused organs are also useful in examining paracrine mediators. These systems allow an investigator to collect and assay small volumes of venous perfusate for the agent in question.

One GI peptide, somatostatin, functions physiologically as a paracrine to inhibit gastrin release and gastric acid secretion. Somatostatin was first isolated from the hypothalamus as a growth hormone release–inhibitory factor. It has since been shown to exist throughout the gastric and duodenal mucosa and the pancreas in high concentrations and to inhibit the release of all gut hormones. Somatostatin mediates the inhibition of gastrin release occurring when the antral mucosa is acidified. Somatostatin also directly inhibits acid secretion from the parietal cells and the release of histamine from ECL cells. These are important physiologic actions of this peptide.

Histamine is a second important paracrine agent. Produced in ECL cells by the decarboxylation of histidine, histamine is released by gastrin and then stimulates acid secretion from the gastric parietal cells. Histamine also potentiates the action of gastrin and ACh on acid secretion. This is why the histamine H_2 receptor–blocking drugs, such as cimetidine (Tagamet) and ranitidine (Zantac), are effective inhibitors of acid secretion regardless of the stimulus. Although parietal cells respond directly to gastrin, released histamine accounts for most of the stimulation of acid secretion by this hormone.

CLINICAL APPLICATIONS

Non–beta cell tumors of the pancreas or duodenal tumors may produce gastrin and continually release it into the blood. This disease is known as *gastrinoma* or *Zollinger-Ellison syndrome*. The tumors are small and difficult to define and resect; if metastasizing, they grow slowly. Gastrin is released from these tumors at a high spontaneous rate that is not altered by feeding. The hypergastrinemia results in hypersecretion of gastric acid through two mechanisms. First, the trophic action of gastrin leads to increased parietal cell mass and acid secretory capacity. Second, increased serum gastrin levels constantly stimulate secretion from the hyperplastic mucosa. The complications of this disease—fulminant peptic ulceration, diarrhea, steatorrhea, and hypokalemia—are caused by the presence of large amounts of acid in the small bowel. The continual presence of acid in the duodenum overwhelms the neutralizing ability of the pancreas, erodes the mucosa, and produces ulcers. In large amounts, gastrin inhibits absorption of fluid and electrolytes by the intestine and thereby adds to the large volumes of fluid (up to 10 liters [L]/day) entering the intestine. Increased intestinal transit

probably also contributes to the diarrhea. Steatorrhea is produced by inactivation of pancreatic lipase and precipitation of bile salts at a low luminal pH. Because the tumors are difficult to resect and the clinical manifestations are caused by hypersecretion of gastric acid, the preferred surgical treatment is removal of the target organ (the stomach). Although gastrin levels remain elevated, total gastrectomy stops the ulceration and diarrhea. This disease also may be treated nonsurgically with some of the powerful new drugs that inhibit acid secretion (see Chapter 8).

The only other clinical condition attributed to the overproduction of a GI peptide concerns VIP. Pancreatic cholera, or watery diarrhea syndrome, is a frequently lethal disease resulting from the secretion of a peptide by a pancreatic islet cell tumor. This peptide is a potent stimulus for intestinal secretion of the fluid and electrolytes that produce the copious diarrhea. VIP has been identified in both the tumor tissue and the serum of these patients. The ability of VIP to stimulate cholera-like fluid secretion from the intestine indicates that it is responsible for this disease.

CLINICAL TESTS

Gastrin is routinely measured by radioimmunoassay in clinical laboratories. Normal serum gastrin values must be set by each laboratory for its particular assay. If the normal mean serum gastrin concentration is taken as 50 picograms (pg)/milliliter (mL), serum gastrin in fasting patients with gastrinoma usually exceeds 200 pg/mL. The degree of overlap between patients with gastrinoma and those with ordinary duodenal ulcer disease means that specific tests are required to diagnose the gastrinoma.

The tests most widely used in the evaluation of hypergastrinemia include stimulation with protein meals, intravenous calcium infusion, and secretin infusion. Patients with Zollinger-Ellison syndrome may not release gastrin in detectable amounts in

response to food. The reason may be the low pH of gastric contents that is caused by ongoing acid secretion stimulated by preexisting high serum gastrin levels. Acid in the antrum inhibits gastrin release, and any gastrin that could be released would be difficult to detect against the already high serum levels.

Patients with gastrinoma may have an exaggerated acid secretory response to calcium infusions that is caused by the release of gastrin from tumor tissue. This test is run by infusing 5 milligrams (mg) of ionizable calcium/kilogram (kg)/hour as calcium gluconate for 3 hours while simultaneously measuring acid secretion and collecting blood samples at hourly intervals for gastrin determination. Peak gastrin responses are usually obtained 3 hours after

Continued

CLINICAL TESTS—cont'd

calcium infusion is begun. In most patients with gastrinoma, serum gastrin concentrations will at least double, so the gastrin values will be more than 500 pg/mL. Patients with ordinary ulcer disease may show moderate increases in serum gastrin with calcium infusion, but absolute gastrin values after stimulation seldom exceed 200 to 300 pg/mL.

The most specific and easiest test to administer for gastrinoma is secretin injection. Secretin inhibits antral gastrin release, yet it stimulates tumor gastrin release in almost all patients with gastrinoma. Secretin (1 unit [U]/kg) is given as a rapid intravenous injection and causes a peak increase in serum gastrin 5 to 10 minutes later. In a patient with definitely increased basal serum gastrin and acid hypersecretion, a doubling of serum gastrin at 5 to 10 minutes strongly indicates the presence of a gastrinoma.

SUMMARY

1. The functions of the GI tract are regulated by mediators acting as hormones (endocrines), paracrines, or neurocrines.
2. Two chemically related families of peptides are responsible for much of the regulation of GI function. These are gastrin/CCK peptides and a second group containing secretin, VIP, GIP, and glucagon.
3. The GI hormones are located in endocrine cells scattered throughout the mucosa and released by chemicals in food, neural activity, or physical distention.
4. The GI peptides have many pharmacologic actions, but only a few of these are physiologically significant.
5. Gastrin, CCK, secretin, GIP, and motilin are important GI hormones.
6. Somatostatin and histamine have important functions as paracrine agents.
7. VIP, bombesin (or GRP), and the enkephalins are released from nerves and mediate many important functions of the digestive tract.

KEY WORDS AND CONCEPTS

Endocrines/hormones	Gastric inhibitory peptide
Paracrines	Motilin
Neurocrines	Gastrin II
Acetylcholine	Vasoactive intestinal
Secretin	peptide
Gastrin	Glucagon
Cholecystokinin	Enteroglucagon
Enterogastrone	G-Gly

CCK-B receptor	Peptide YY
Amine precursor uptake decarboxylation	Glucagon-like peptide-1
	Somatostatin
Enterochromaffin-like cells	Histamine
Pancreatic polypeptide	

SUGGESTED READINGS

Chao C, Hellmich MR: Gastrointestinal peptides: gastrin, cholecystokinin, somatostatin, and ghrelin. In Johnson LR, editor: ed 5, *Physiology of the Gastrointestinal Tract*, vol 1, San Diego, 2012, Elsevier.

Gomez GA, Englander EW, Greeley GH Jr: Postpyloric gastrointestinal peptides. In Johnson LR, editor: ed 5, *Physiology of the Gastrointestinal Tract*, vol 1, San Diego, 2012, Elsevier.

Johnson LR: Regulation of gastrointestinal mucosal growth. In Johnson LR, editor: *Physiology of the Gastrointestinal Tract*, ed 3, New York, 1994, Raven Press.

Makhlouf GM, editor: *Handbook of Physiology, Section 6: The Gastrointestinal System, vol. 2: Neural and Endocrine Biology*, Bethesda, MD, 1989, American Physiological Society.

Modlin IM, Sachs G: *Acid Related Diseases*, Milan, 1998, Schnetztor Verlag Gmbh D-Konstanz.

Pearse AGE, Takor T: Embryology of the diffuse neuroendocrine system and its relationship to the common peptides, *Fed Proc* 38:2288–2294, 1979.

Rozengurt E, Walsh JH: Gastrin, CCK, signaling, and cancer, *Annu Rev Physiol* 63:49–76, 2001.

Solcia E, Capella C, Buffa R, et al: Endocrine cells of the digestive system. In Johnson LR, editor: *Physiology of the Gastrointestinal Tract*, ed 2, New York, 1987, Raven Press.

Walsh JH: Gastrointestinal hormones. In Johnson LR, editor: *Physiology of the Gastrointestinal Tract*, ed 3, New York, 1994, Raven Press.

Walsh JH, Grossman MI: Gastrin, *N Engl J Med* 292:1324–1332, 1337–1384, 1975.

Walsh JH, Grossman MI: The Zollinger-Ellison syndrome, *Gastroenterology* 65:140–165, 1973.

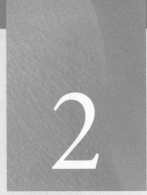

2 REGULATION: NERVES AND SMOOTH MUSCLE

OBJECTIVES

- Understand the anatomy and functions of the enteric nervous system and its relationship with the parasympathetic and sympathetic systems.
- Describe the anatomy and types of contractions of smooth muscle cells.
- Explain the role of calcium ion in the contraction and relaxation of smooth muscle cells.
- Understand the roles of the interstitial cells of Cajal and slow waves in the contraction of smooth muscle cells.

Secretory, motility, and absorptive functions of the gastrointestinal (GI) system are integrated to digest food and absorb nutrients and to maintain homeostasis between meals. This integration is mediated by regulatory systems that monitor events within the body (primarily the GI tract) and in the external environment. In Chapter 1, the important mediators released from endocrine, paracrine, and neurocrine cells are discussed. In this chapter, the role of the nervous system is considered in more detail.

Although the regulatory systems act to integrate the activities of the GI system, most secretory, absorptive, and muscle cells possess intrinsic activities that give them a degree of autonomy. Thus function arises out of the interaction of regulatory systems and local intrinsic properties. The basic properties and intrinsic activities of each type of secretory and absorptive cell are discussed in separate chapters that deal with the secretion and absorption of specific chemicals. The basic properties and intrinsic activities of the smooth muscle cells are discussed in this chapter.

ANATOMY OF THE AUTONOMIC NERVOUS SYSTEM

The GI tract is innervated by the **autonomic nervous system** (ANS). It is called the ANS because, under normal circumstances, people neither are conscious of its activities nor exert any willful control over them. The ANS can be divided into the extrinsic nervous system and the intrinsic, or enteric, nervous system.

The **extrinsic nervous system** is in turn divided into parasympathetic and sympathetic branches (Fig. 2-1). **Parasympathetic innervation** is supplied primarily by the vagus and pelvic nerves. Long preganglionic axons arise from cell bodies within the medulla of the brain and the sacral region of the spinal cord. These preganglionic nerves enter the various organs of the GI tract, where they synapse mainly with cells of the enteric nervous system (Fig. 2-2). In addition, these same nerve bundles contain many afferent nerves whose receptors lie within the various tissues of the gut. These nerves project to the brain and spinal cord to provide sensory input for integration. Approximately 75% of the fibers within the vagus nerve are afferent. Thus information can be relayed from the GI tract to the medulla and integrated, and a message can be sent back to the tract that may influence motility, secretion, or the release of a hormone. These long or **vagovagal reflexes** play important roles in regulating GI functions.

Sympathetic innervation is supplied by nerves that run between the spinal cord and the prevertebral ganglia and between these ganglia and the organs of the gut. Preganglionic efferent fibers arise within the spinal cord and end in the prevertebral ganglia. Postganglionic fibers from these ganglia then innervate

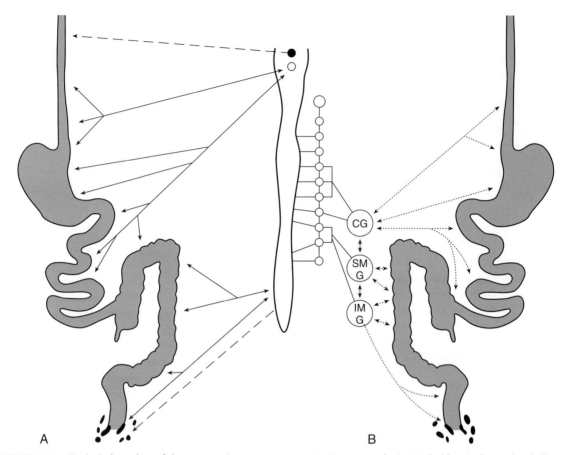

FIGURE 2-1 ■ Extrinsic branches of the autonomic nervous system. **A,** Parasympathetic. *Dashed lines* indicate the cholinergic innervation of striated muscle in the esophagus and external anal sphincter. *Solid lines* indicate the afferent and preganglionic efferent innervation of the rest of the gastrointestinal tract. **B,** Sympathetic. *Solid lines* denote the afferent and preganglionic efferent connections between the spinal cord and the prevertebral ganglia. *Dashed lines* indicate the afferent and postganglionic efferent innervation. CG, celiac ganglion; IMG, inferior mesenteric ganglion; SMG, superior mesenteric ganglion.

primarily the elements of the enteric nervous system (see Fig. 2-1). Few fibers end directly on secretory, absorptive, or muscle cells. Afferent fibers also are present within the sympathetic division. These nerves project back to the prevertebral ganglia and/or the spinal cord. Thus an abundance of sensory information also is available via these nerves.

Elements of the **intrinsic,** or **enteric, nervous system** are grouped into several anatomically distinct networks, of which the **myenteric** and **submucosal plexuses** (see Fig. 2-2) are the most prominent. These plexuses consist of nerve cell bodies, axons, dendrites, and nerve endings. Processes from the neurons of the

plexuses do not just innervate target cells such as smooth muscle, secretory cells, and absorptive cells. They also connect to sensory receptors and interdigitate with processes from other neurons located both inside and outside the plexus. Thus pathways within the enteric nervous system can be multisynaptic, and integration of activities can take place entirely within the enteric nervous system (see Fig. 2-2), as well as in the ganglia of the extrinsic nerves, the spinal cord, and the brainstem.

Many chemicals serve as **neurocrines** within the ANS. Several of these chemicals have been localized within specific pathways, and a few have defined

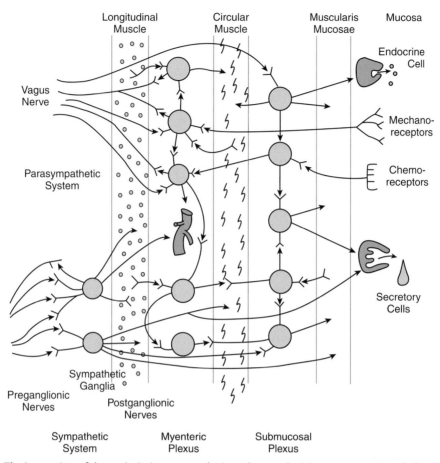

FIGURE 2-2 ■ The integration of the extrinsic (parasympathetic and sympathetic) nervous system with the enteric (myenteric and submucosal plexuses) nervous system. The preganglionic fibers of the parasympathetic synapse with ganglion cells located in the enteric nervous system. Their cell bodies, in turn, send signals to smooth muscle, secretory, and endocrine cells. They also receive information from receptors located in the mucosa and in the smooth muscle that is relayed to higher centers via vagal afferents. This may result in vagovagal (long) reflexes. Postganglionic efferent fibers from the sympathetic ganglia innervate the elements of the enteric system, but they also innervate smooth muscle, blood vessels, and secretory cells directly. The enteric nervous system relays information up and down the length of the gastrointestinal tract, and this may result in short or intrinsic reflexes. *(Reprinted with permission from Johnson LR. Essential Medical Physiology, 3rd ed. Philadelphia, Academic Press, 2003.)*

physiologic roles. Most of the extrinsic, preganglionic, efferent fibers contain **acetylcholine** (ACh). This transmitter exerts its action on neurons contained within the prevertebral ganglia and enteric nervous system. **Norepinephrine** is found in many nerve endings of the postganglionic efferent nerves of the sympathetic nervous system. This transmitter also exerts its effects primarily on neurons of the enteric nervous system. Within the enteric nervous system, ACh, **serotonin, vasoactive intestinal peptide** (VIP),

nitric oxide (NO), and **somatostatin** have been localized to interneurons. ACh and the tachykinins (TKs) (e.g., **substance P**) have been localized to nerves that are excitatory to the muscle; VIP and NO have been localized to inhibitory nerves to the muscle. In many instances, more than one transmitter can be localized to the same nerve. The goals of mapping neural circuits within the extrinsic and enteric nervous system and elucidating their functions are far from complete.

NEUROHUMORAL REGULATION OF GASTROINTESTINAL FUNCTION

Although it is convenient to discuss the ANS and the endocrine/paracrine systems separately, it is important to understand that they do not function independently of one another. Rather, the regulatory systems interact to control secretion, absorption, and motility. Specific examples of such regulation are given in subsequent chapters (see Figs. 8-10 and 9-7 for examples). The targets, be they secretory, absorptive, or smooth muscle cells, have a certain resting output that is modulated by both neurally released chemicals and humorally delivered chemicals. These chemicals are released from nerve endings and glandular cells in response to various stimuli that act on specific receptors. The sources of these stimuli can be either in the environment or within the body. For example, seeing or smelling appetizing food alters many aspects of GI function, as does the presence of many foodstuffs and products of digestion within the lumen of the stomach and intestine. In many cases, the stimuli result from the secretory and motor functions of the target cells themselves. Whatever their source, these stimuli initiate inputs that are integrated in the neural and endocrine systems to produce outputs that appropriately regulate the functions of the target cells.

ANATOMY OF THE SMOOTH MUSCLE CELL

The contractile tissue of the GI tract is made up of **smooth muscle cells,** except in the pharynx, orad third of the esophagus, and external anal sphincter. The smooth muscle cells found in each region of the GI tract exhibit functional and structural differences. These special features are considered in subsequent chapters. However, certain basic properties are common to all smooth muscle cells. The cells, which are 4 to 10 micrometers (μm) wide and 50 to 200 μm long, are small when compared with skeletal muscle cells. A distinguishing feature of these cells is that the contractile elements are not arranged in orderly sarcomeres as in skeletal muscle (Fig. 2-3). Thus the cells have no striations. Many of the contractile proteins found in striated muscle also exist in smooth muscle, although they differ in isoform and in relative amounts. Actin,

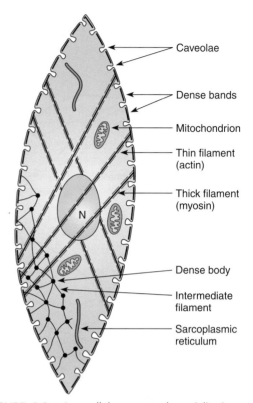

FIGURE 2-3 ■ Intracellular structural specializations of a smooth muscle cell. N, nucleus. *(Adapted from Schiller LR: Motor function of the stomach. In Sleisenger MH, Fordtran JS [eds]: Gastrointestinal Disease. Philadelphia, Saunders, 1983.)*

along with tropomyosin, is the main constituent of thin filaments, whereas myosin is the main constituent of thick filaments. Compared with skeletal muscle, smooth muscle contains less myosin, much more actin, and little if any troponin. The apparent ratio of thin to thick filaments in smooth muscles is 12:1 to 18:1, rather than 2:1 as in skeletal muscle. In addition to the thick and thin filaments, smooth muscle cells contain a third network of filaments that form an internal "skeleton." These intermediate filaments, along with their associated dense bodies, may serve as anchor points for the contractile filaments and may modulate contractile activity.

Smooth muscle cells of the GI tract are grouped into branching bundles, or **fasciae,** that are surrounded by connective tissue sheets. These fasciae, organized into muscular coats, can serve as the effector units because smooth muscle cells of the gut are mostly

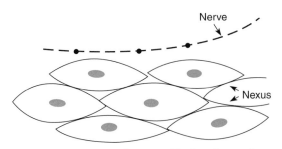

FIGURE 2-4 ■ Anatomic features of "unitary" smooth muscle. Neurotransmitter is released from varicosities along the nerve trunk. Other chemicals arrive via endocrine and paracrine routes. The influence of these substances on one muscle cell is then transmitted to other cells via nexuses.

of the "unitary" type (Fig. 2-4). Individual cells are functionally coupled to one another so that the contractions of a bundle of muscle are synchronous. In most tissues, this coupling is the result of actual fusion of apposing membranes in the form of gap junctions or nexuses. These junctions serve as areas of low resistance for the spread of excitation from one cell to another. Not every smooth muscle cell is innervated. Nerve axons enter the muscle bundles and release neurotransmitters from swellings along their length.

These swellings usually are some distance from the muscle cells so that no discrete neuromuscular junctions exist. Thus the neurotransmitters probably act on only a few of the muscle cells or on interstitial cells of Cajal (ICCs), which in turn form junctions with muscle cells. The influence of the transmitters must then be communicated from one smooth muscle cell to the next.

SMOOTH MUSCLE CONTRACTION

The time course of contractions among smooth muscles in the GI tract has remarkable heterogeneity. Some muscles, such as those found in the body of the esophagus, small bowel, and gastric antrum, contract and relax in a matter of seconds (**phasic contractions**). Other smooth muscles, such as those found in the lower esophageal sphincter, orad stomach, and ileocecal and internal anal sphincters, show sustained contractions that last from minutes to hours. These muscles exhibit what are called **tonic contractions.** As discussed in subsequent chapters, the type of contraction, whether phasic or tonic, is governed by the

smooth muscle cells themselves or by ICCs in association with smooth muscle cells. It does not depend on neural or hormonal input. Neurocrines, endocrines, and paracrines are important because they modulate the basic contractile activity, so that the amplitude of the contractions of phasic muscles varies and the tone of the tonic muscles increases or decreases.

As in striated muscle, contractile activity of smooth muscle, especially those muscles that contract phasically, is modulated by fluctuating levels of free intracellular **calcium** (Ca^{2+}). At low levels (less than 10^{-7} molar [M]) of Ca^{2+}, interaction of the contractile proteins does not occur. At higher levels of Ca^{2+}, proteins interact and contractions occur. The prevailing theory to explain how Ca^{2+} brings about contraction is that the Ca^{2+}, combined with the Ca^{2+}-binding protein calmodulin, activates a protein kinase that brings about the specific phosphorylation of one of the components of myosin (Fig. 2-5). Myosin in its phosphorylated form then interacts with actin to cause contraction, which is fueled by the splitting of **adenosine triphosphate** (ATP). When the intracellular levels of Ca^{2+} fall, the myosin is dephosphorylated by a specific phosphatase. This leads to a cessation of the interaction between the contractile proteins, and muscle relaxation occurs. In smooth muscles that contract tonically, the exact mechanism for the maintenance of tone is not known. What is known is that tone can be maintained at low levels of phosphorylation of myosin and of ATP utilization. In addition, it is becoming apparent that smooth muscle contraction is regulated not only by levels of Ca^{2+} but also by processes that regulate the activity of the phosphatase(s) that dephosphorylates myosin, thereby altering the Ca^{2+} sensitivity of the contractile process.

The exact source of the Ca^{2+} that participates in the contractile process is not certain and appears to vary from one muscle to another. In many muscles (e.g., muscle from the body of the esophagus), Ca^{2+} enters the cells from the extracellular fluid or from pools of Ca^{2+} that are tightly bound to the smooth muscle cell membranes or contained in caveolae (see Fig. 2-3). Influx of Ca^{2+} from these sites is regulated by permeability changes of the membrane that also cause characteristic electrical activities (see the following paragraph). In other muscles (e.g., muscle from the lower esophageal sphincter), Ca^{2+} is sequestered in

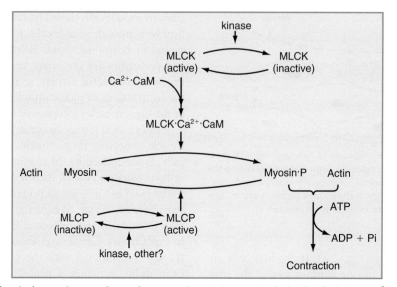

FIGURE 2-5 ■ Biochemical events in smooth muscle contraction. An increase in the levels of calcium (Ca^{2+}) activates the enzyme myosin light chain kinase (MLCK), which phosphorylates myosin. Phosphorylated myosin (Myosin P) interacts with actin to cause muscle contraction and adenosine triphosphate (ATP) consumption. When Ca^{2+} levels fall, the kinase becomes inactive, and the activity of myosin light chain phosphatase (MLCP) dominates. Myosin P is dephosphorylated, and the muscle relaxes. The activities of both MLCK and MLCP can be modulated by kinases and/or second messengers to influence calcium sensitivity of the contractile process. ADP, adenosine diphosphate; CaM, calmodulin; Pi, inorganic phosphate.

intracellular structures called the *sarcoplasmic reticulum* (see Fig. 2-4) and is released in response to electrical events of the plasma membrane or to agonist-induced increases in inositol triphosphate, or to both. In addition to these sources for Ca^{2+}, mechanisms also exist for the expulsion of Ca^{2+} from the cells and for reuptake into the sarcoplasmic reticulum.

Increases in free intracellular Ca^{2+} most often are related to electrical activities of the smooth muscle cell membranes. In phasically active muscle, Ca^{2+} enters the cell by way of voltage-dependent Ca^{2+} channels. When these channels are activated, rapid transients in membrane potential occur; these are called **action** or **spike potentials** (see Fig. 5-6). In many physically active muscles, these spike potentials do not arise from a stable resting membrane potential. Rather, they are superimposed on relatively slow (3 to 12 cycles/minute) but regular oscillations in membrane potential.

These potential changes, called **slow waves,** do not in themselves cause significant contractions. They set the timing, however, for when spike potentials can occur because spikes are seen only during the peak of depolarization of the slow wave.

The genesis of slow waves appears to lie in complex interactions among smooth muscle cells and specialized cells called **interstitial cells of Cajal** (ICCs) (Fig. 2-6). In all regions of the GI tract from which slow waves are recorded, ICCs are present and are connected to one another to form a three-dimensional network within and/or between the smooth muscle layers. These cells not only communicate with one another but also form gap junctions with smooth muscle cells. Some ICCs appear to be interposed between enteric nerve endings and smooth muscle cells and may be involved in neural modulation of smooth muscle activity rather than in slow wave generation. Isolated ICCs exhibit membrane properties that could provide the pacemaker activity responsible for the generation of slow waves. This activity spreads into and affects the smooth muscle cells. Both slow waves and spike potentials are recorded from smooth muscle cells that are coupled to ICCs, but slow waves are absent from intestinal smooth muscle devoid of ICCs (see Fig. 2-6).

Slow waves are extremely regular and are only minimally influenced by neural or hormonal activities, although they are influenced by body temperature and metabolic activity. The higher the activity,

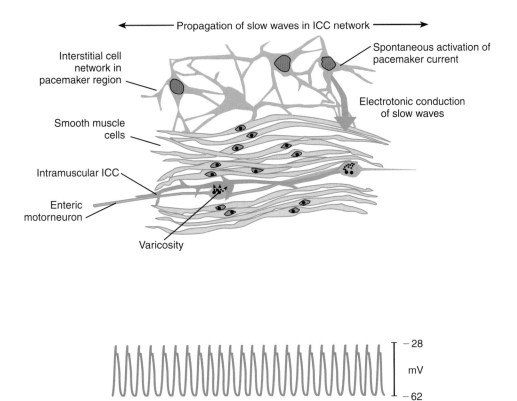

FIGURE 2-6 ■ **Top,** Interactions among interstitial cells of Cajal (ICCs), smooth muscle cells, and nerves. Pacemaker current leading to slow waves appears to originate in the ICC network. Slow waves actively propagate within the ICC network and are passively conducted into the smooth muscle. Other ICCs appear to be interposed between nerve endings and smooth muscle cells; they may be involved in neuromodulation. **Bottom,** Recordings of electrical activity from the small intestine of a normal mouse (A) and a mouse deficient in ICCs (B). Note the absence of slow waves in B. *(Modified from Horowitz B, Ward SM, Sanders KM: Cellular and molecular basis for electrical rhythmicity in gastrointestinal muscles. Annu Rev Physiol 61:19-43, 1999.)*

the higher is the frequency of slow waves. Conversely, the occurrence of spike potentials depends heavily on neural and hormonal activities.

An excitatory endocrine, paracrine, or neurocrine acts on a receptor on the smooth muscle cell membrane to induce spike potentials in those cells and in adjacent cells that are coupled to one another. The spike potentials lead to an increase in intercellular free Ca^{2+} levels. The Ca^{2+} then acts via myosin light chain kinase to induce **contraction.** In contrast, an inhibitory mediator acts with its receptor on that same membrane. In this case, however, the response is an inhibition of spike potentials or a hyperpolarization of the cell membrane or both. This results in a decrease in intracellular free Ca^{2+} and subsequent **relaxation.** In addition, evidence indicates that activation of cell receptors also can modulate contractile activity through mechanisms not involving the Ca^{2+}-myosin phosphorylation pathway. Whatever the mechanism, it is the interplay of these excitatory and inhibitory mediators on the basal activity of the muscle that determines the motility functions of the various organs of the gut.

SUMMARY

1. The regulation of GI function results from an interplay of neural and hormonal influences on effector cells that have intrinsic activities.
2. The GI tract is innervated by the ANS, which is composed of nerves that are extrinsic and nerves that are intrinsic to the tract.
3. Extrinsic nerves are distributed to the GI tract through both parasympathetic and sympathetic pathways.
4. Intrinsic nerves are grouped into several nerve plexuses, of which the myenteric and submucosal plexuses are the most prominent. Nerves in the plexuses receive input from receptors within the GI tract and from extrinsic nerves. This input can be integrated within the intrinsic nerves such that coordinated activities can be effected.
5. ACh is one of the major excitatory neurotransmitters, and NO and VIP are two of the major inhibitory neurotransmitters at effector cells. Serotonin and somatostatin are two important neurotransmitters of intrinsic interneurons.
6. Striated muscle comprises the musculature of the pharynx, the oral half of the esophagus, and the external anal sphincter. Smooth muscle makes up the musculature of the rest of the GI tract.
7. Adjacent smooth muscle cells are electrically coupled to one another and contract synchronously when stimulated. Some smooth muscles contract tonically, whereas others contract phasically.
8. In phasically active muscle, stimulation induces a rise in intracellular Ca^{2+}, which in turn induces phosphorylation of the 20,000-dalton light chain of myosin. ATP is split, and the muscle contracts as the phosphorylated myosin (myosin P) interacts with actin. Ca^{2+} levels fall, myosin is dephosphorylated, and relaxation occurs. In tonically active muscles, contraction can be maintained at low levels of phosphorylation and ATP utilization.
9. Periodic membrane depolarizations and repolarizations, called slow waves, are major determinants of the phasic nature of contraction. Slow wave activity results from ionic currents initiated through the interactions of the ICCs with smooth muscle cells.

KEY WORDS AND CONCEPTS

Autonomic nervous system

Extrinsic nervous system

Parasympathetic innervation

Vagovagal reflexes

Sympathetic innervation

Intrinsic/enteric nervous system

Myenteric/submucosal plexuses

Neurocrines

Acetylcholine

Norepinephrine

Serotonin

Vasoactive intestinal peptide

Nitric oxide

Somatostatin

Substance P

Smooth muscle cells

Fasciae

Phasic contractions

Tonic contractions

Calcium

Adenosine triphosphate

Action/spike potentials

Slow waves

Interstitial cells of Cajal

Contraction

Relaxation

SUGGESTED READINGS

Bitar KN, Gilmont RR, Raghavan S, Somara S: Cellular physiology of gastrointestinal smooth muscle. In Johnson LR, editor: ed 5, *Physiology of the Gastrointestinal Tract*, vol 1, San Diego, 2012, Elsevier.

Murphy RA: Muscle in the walls of hollow organs. In Berne RM, Levy MN, editors: *Principles of Physiology*, ed 3, St. Louis, 2000, Mosby.

Pfitzer G: Signal transduction in smooth muscle. Invited review: regulation of myosin phosphorylation in smooth muscle, *J Appl Physiol* 91:497–503, 2001.

Roman C, Gonella J: Extrinsic control of digestive tract motility. In Johnson LR, editor: ed 2, *Physiology of the Gastrointestinal Tract*, vol 1, New York, 1987, Raven Press.

Sanders KM, Koh SD, Ward SM: Organization and electrophysiology of interstitial cells of Cajal and smooth muscle cells in the gastrointestinal tract. In Johnson LR, editor: ed 5, *Physiology of the Gastrointestinal Tract*, vol 1, San Diego, 2012, Elsevier.

Wood JD: Integrative functions of the enteric nervous system. In Johnson LR, editor: ed 5, *Physiology of the Gastrointestinal Tract*, vol 1, San Diego, 2012, Elsevier.

3   SWALLOWING

OBJECTIVES

- Describe the oral and pharyngeal events taking place during a swallow.
- Describe the pressures within the esophagus and oral stomach at rest and during a swallow.
- Explain the regulation involved during a swallow, including its initiation and peristalsis through the esophagus.
- Understand the process of receptive relaxation of the oral stomach, its function, and regulation.
- Understand gastric esophageal reflux disease (GERD) and its causes.

Swallowing consists of chewing, a pharyngeal phase, movement of material through the esophagus, and the relaxation of the stomach to receive the ingested material. Swallowing is almost purely a motility function. Digestion and absorption are minimal, in part because transport of the bolus into the stomach takes only seconds.

CHEWING

Chewing has three major functions: (1) it facilitates swallowing by reducing the size of ingested particles and thus also prevents damage to the lining of the pharynx and esophagus; (2) it mixes food with saliva, which exposes the food to digestive enzymes and lubricates it; (3) it increases the surface area of ingested material and thereby increases the rate at which it can be digested.

The act of chewing is both voluntary and involuntary, and most of the time it proceeds by reflexes void of conscious input. The **chewing reflex** is initiated by food in the mouth that inhibits muscles of mastication and causes the jaw to drop. A subsequent stretch reflex of the jaw muscles produces a contraction that automatically raises the jaw and closes the teeth on the bolus of food. Compression of the bolus on the mucosal surface of the mouth inhibits the jaw muscles to repeat the process.

PHARYNGEAL PHASE

Normally liquids are propelled immediately from the mouth to the **oropharynx** and are swallowed. Swallowing is initiated by propulsion of material into the oropharynx primarily by movements of the **tongue.** The portion of solid material to be swallowed is separated from other material in the mouth so it lies in a chamber created by placing the tip of the tongue against the hard palate (Fig. 3-1, *A*). The material is propelled by elevation and retraction of the tongue against the palate. As the material passes from the **oral cavity** into the oropharynx, the **nasopharynx** is closed by movement of the soft palate and contraction of the superior constrictor muscles of the pharynx (Fig. 3-1, *B*). Simultaneously, respiration is inhibited, and contraction of the laryngeal muscles closes the **glottis** and raises the **larynx.** The bolus is propelled through the pharynx by a **peristaltic contraction** that begins in the superior constrictor and progresses through the middle and inferior constrictor muscles of the **pharynx** (Fig. 3-1, *C*). These contractions, along with relaxation of the **upper esophageal sphincter** (UES), propel the bolus into the esophagus (Fig. 3-1, *D*).

21

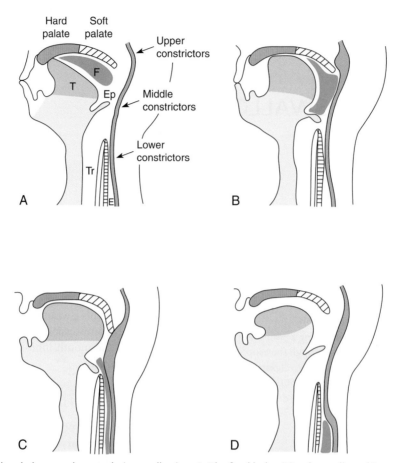

FIGURE 3-1 ■ Oral and pharyngeal events during swallowing. **A,** The food bolus (F) to be swallowed is propelled into the pharynx by placement of the tongue (T) on the roof of the hard palate. E, esophagus; Ep, epiglottis; Tr, trachea. **B,** Further propulsion is caused by movement of the more distal regions of the tongue against the palate. Contraction of the upper constrictors of the pharynx and movement of the soft palate separate the oropharynx from the nasopharynx. **C,** Propulsion through the upper esophageal sphincter is accomplished by contraction of the middle and lower constrictors of the pharynx and by relaxation of the cricopharyngeal muscle. Upward movement of the glottis and downward movement of the epiglottis seal off the trachea. **D,** The bolus is now in the esophagus and is propelled into the stomach by a peristaltic contraction.

The oral and pharyngeal phases of swallowing are rapid, taking less than 1 second. Swallowing can be initiated voluntarily, but these efforts fail unless something, at least a small amount of saliva, triggers the swallowing reflex. Once initiated, however, swallowing proceeds as a coordinated involuntary reflex. Coordination is central in origin, and an area within the reticular formation of the brainstem has been identified as the **swallowing center.** Afferent impulses from the pharynx are directed toward this center, which serves to coordinate the activity of other areas of the brain such as the nuclei of the trigeminal, facial, and hypoglossal nerves, as well as the nucleus ambiguus (Fig. 3-2). Efferent impulses from the center are distributed to the pharynx via nerves from the nucleus ambiguus. The impulses appear to be sequential, so the pharyngeal musculature is activated in a proximal-to-distal manner. This sequencing accounts for the peristaltic nature of the pharyngeal contractions. The center also appears to interact with other areas of the brain involved with respiration and speech. Injury to the swallowing center produces abnormalities in the pharyngeal component of swallowing.

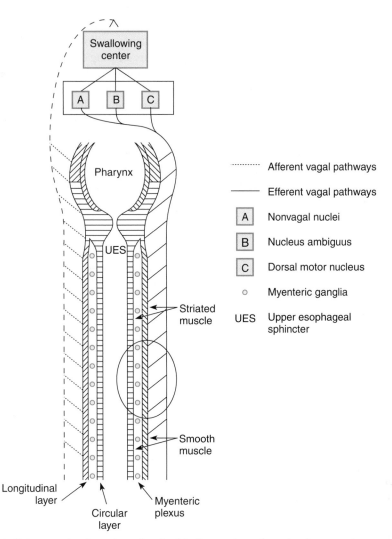

FIGURE 3-2 ■ Control of pharyngeal and esophageal peristalsis. Sensory input from the pharynx activates an area in the medulla (the swallowing center). This center serves to coordinate activation of the vagal nuclei with other centers such as the respiratory centers. Muscles of the pharynx and striated areas of the esophagus are activated by the center via the nucleus ambiguus. Areas of the smooth muscle are activated via the dorsal motor nucleus. Peristalsis results from sequential activation of the muscles of the pharynx and esophagus by sequential neural impulses from the center. The *area enclosed within the circle* is shown in more detail in Figure 3-4.

ESOPHAGEAL PERISTALSIS

The **esophagus** propels material from the pharynx to the stomach. This propulsion is accomplished by coordinated contractions of the muscular layers of the body of the esophagus. Because a large segment of the esophagus is located in the thorax, where the pressure is lower than in the pharynx and stomach, the esophagus also must withstand the entry of air and gastric contents. The barrier functions of the esophagus are accomplished by the presence of sphincters at each end of the organ.

Anatomically the esophageal muscle is arranged in two layers: an inner layer with the muscle fibers organized in a circular axis and an outer layer with the fibers organized in a longitudinal axis. The UES consists of a thickening of the circular muscle and can be identified anatomically as the cricopharyngeal muscle. This muscle, like the musculature of the proximal third of the esophageal body, is striated. The distal third of the esophagus is composed of smooth muscle; although the terminal 1 to 2 centimeters (cm) of the musculature acts as a **lower esophageal sphincter** (LES), no separate sphincter muscle can be identified anatomically. The middle third of the body of the esophagus is composed of a mixture of muscle types with a descending transition from striated to smooth fibers.

The events that occur in the esophagus between and during swallowing are often monitored by placing pressure-sensing devices at various levels in the esophageal lumen. Such devices indicate that between swallows, both the UES and the LES are closed and the body of the esophagus is flaccid (Fig. 3-3, *A*). In the region of the UES, pressure is as much as 60 millimeters of mercury (mm Hg) higher than that in the pharynx or body of the esophagus. A zone of elevated pressure also is found at the LES. The length of this zone may range from several millimeters to a few centimeters, and the pressure may be 20 to 40 mm Hg

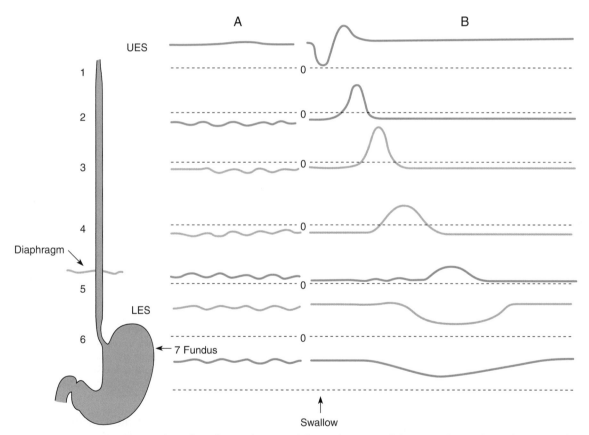

FIGURE 3-3 ▪ Manometric recordings from the esophagus and the orad portion of the stomach. Intraluminal pressures from the upper esophageal sphincter (UES), four areas of the esophagus, the lower esophageal sphincter (LES), and the gastric fundus are shown. **A,** Between swallows, both the upper and the lower sphincters are closed, as indicated by the greater than atmospheric pressures recorded there. Pressures in the body of the esophagus reflect intrathoracic or intra-abdominal pressures. Pressures in the fundus reflect intra-abdominal pressure plus tonic contractions of the fundus. **B,** On swallowing, the upper sphincter relaxes before passage of the bolus. After bolus passage it contracts, followed by a peristaltic contraction in the body of the esophagus. To allow passage of the bolus into the stomach, the lower sphincter and the orad stomach relax before the peristaltic contraction reaches them.

higher than on either side. Pressures in the body of the esophagus are similar to those within the body cavity in which the esophagus lies. In the thorax the pressures are subatmospheric and vary with respiration; they drop with inspiration and rise with expiration. These fluctuations in pressure with respiration reverse below the diaphragm, and intraluminal esophageal pressure reflects intra-abdominal pressure, which is slightly higher than atmospheric pressure.

During a swallow the sphincters and the body of the esophagus act in a coordinated manner (Fig. 3-3, *B*). Shortly before the distal pharyngeal muscles contract, the UES opens. Once the bolus passes, the sphincter closes and assumes its resting tone. The body of the esophagus undergoes a peristaltic contraction.

This contraction begins just below the UES and occurs sequentially at progressively more distal segments to give the appearance of a contractile wave moving toward the stomach. After the contractile sequence passes, the esophageal muscle becomes flaccid again. Shortly before the peristaltic contraction reaches the LES, the sphincter relaxes. After passage of the bolus the sphincter contracts back to its resting level. Compared with the rapid events in the pharynx, esophageal peristalsis is slow. The peristaltic contraction moves down the esophagus at velocities ranging from 2 to 6 cm/second, and it may take the bolus 10 seconds to reach the lower end of the esophagus.

When esophageal peristalsis is preceded by a pharyngeal phase, it is called **primary peristalsis.** Esophageal contractions, however, can occur in the absence of both oral and pharyngeal phases. This phenomenon is called **secondary peristalsis** and is elicited when the esophagus is distended. Secondary peristalsis occurs if the primary contraction fails to empty the esophagus or when gastric contents reflux into the esophagus. Initiation of secondary peristaltic contractions is involuntary and normally is not sensed.

The effect of esophageal peristalsis on bolus transport depends on the physical properties of the bolus. If a person in an upright position swallows a liquid bolus, it actually reaches the stomach several seconds before the peristaltic contraction. Thus although both sphincters must relax to allow transport of all materials, esophageal peristalsis is not always necessary. For most swallowed material, peristaltic contractions are essential for progression to the stomach, and repetitive

secondary contractions are often required to sweep the bolus completely into the stomach.

Control of esophageal peristalsis is complex and not fully understood. Closure of the UES is maintained by the normal elasticity of the sphincteric structures and active contraction of the cricopharyngeal muscle. Relaxation of the UES is coordinated with contraction of the pharyngeal musculature. As the larynx rises during the pharyngeal component of swallowing, the cricopharyngeal area is displaced. This displacement, along with relaxation of the cricopharyngeal muscle, allows the sphincter to open. Relaxation of the cricopharyngeal muscle is brought about by a suppression of nerve impulses from the swallowing center via the activity of the nucleus ambiguus.

Contractions of the body of the esophagus are coordinated by both central and peripheral mechanisms. This region of the esophagus is innervated primarily by the vagus nerves. These nerves are partly of the somatic motor type, arising from the nucleus ambiguus, and partly of the visceral motor type, arising from the dorsal motor nucleus. The somatic motor nerves synapse directly with striated muscle fibers of the esophagus (Fig. 3-4). The visceral motor nerves do not synapse directly with the smooth muscle cells but rather with nerve cell bodies that lie between the longitudinal and circular muscle layers. These local nerves in turn innervate the smooth muscle cells, as well as communicate with one another along the length of the esophagus.

Central control of swallowing originates within the swallowing center, which sends a series of sequential impulses to progressively more distal segments of the esophagus. This sequential activation results in a peristaltic contraction. The central nervous system does not totally control peristalsis, however. In smooth muscle areas of the esophagus, peristalsis can occur after bilateral cervical **vagotomy** (cutting of the vagus nerve). Furthermore, peristalsis can be induced in excised esophagi that have been placed in an organ bath. In these instances, peristalsis must be coordinated by the intrinsic nerve plexuses or the smooth muscle cells themselves.

The presence of secondary peristalsis indicates the importance of afferent input to the central and peripheral mechanisms controlling swallowing. Afferent input provided by distention of the esophagus not only

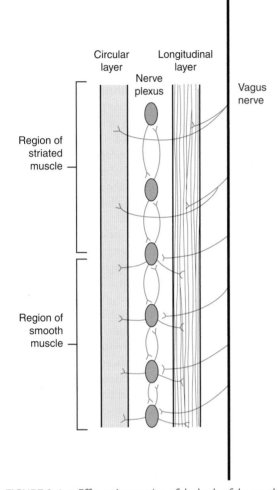

FIGURE 3-4 ■ Efferent innervation of the body of the esophagus. Special visceral somatic fibers directly innervate the striated muscle fibers of the circular and longitudinal muscle layers. Preganglionic fibers from the vagus innervate the ganglion cells of the intrinsic plexus. Fibers from the ganglion cells then innervate the smooth muscle cells of both layers. In addition, the ganglion cells have neural connections with one another.

initiates secondary peristalsis but also affects the intensity of contractions. Variation in the size of the bolus being swallowed leads to a variation in the amplitude of esophageal contraction. Indeed, afferent stimulation appears so important that a peristaltic sequence may not occur unless a bolus is swallowed and elicits afferent stimulation. Conversely, intense afferent stimulation,

such as that provided by inflation of a balloon in the body of the esophagus, can inhibit the progression of peristaltic contractions past the balloon.

Contraction of the LES is regulated by the intrinsic properties of the smooth muscle fibers, as well as by neural and humoral influences. Smooth muscle from this area of the esophagus responds to passive stretching by contracting to oppose the stretch. This response does not depend on nervous activity. Thus the basic tone of the LES may be totally myogenic. Nevertheless, this tone is under several neural and humoral influences. For example, resting tone is increased by cholinergic agonists and by the gastrointestinal hormone gastrin. Sphincteric tone is decreased by agents such as isoproterenol and prostaglandin E_1.

Transient relaxation of the LES during swallowing is mediated through enteric nerves. The enteric inhibitory nerves can be activated by stimulation of the vagus nerve and by distention of the body of the esophagus, thus activating aboral enteric nerves. The neurochemical basis for this response is not known, although roles for both vasoactive intestinal peptide (VIP) and nitric oxide (NO) have been proposed.

RECEPTIVE RELAXATION OF THE STOMACH

Swallowing also involves the stomach. In terms of motility functions, the stomach can be divided into two major areas: the **orad portion,** which consists of the fundus and a portion of the body; and the **caudad portion,** which consists of the distal body and the antrum (Fig. 3-5). These two regions have markedly different patterns of motility that are responsible, in part, for two major functions: accommodation of ingested material during swallowing and regulation of gastric emptying. Accommodation is attributable primarily to activities of the oral region, whereas both regions are involved in the regulation of gastric emptying (see Chapter 4).

During a swallow, the orad region of the stomach relaxes at about the same time as the LES. Intraluminal pressures in both regions fall before arrival of the swallowed bolus because of active relaxation of the smooth muscle in both regions (see Fig. 3-3, B). After passage of the bolus, the pressure in the stomach returns to approximately what it was before the swallow. This

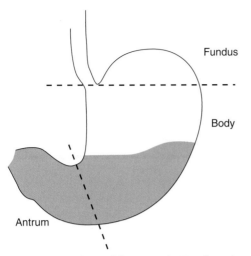

FIGURE 3-5 ■ Divisions of the stomach. For discussions of secretion, the stomach usually is divided into the fundus, body, and antrum. For discussions of motility, it can be divided into an orad area and a caudad area. *Shading* denotes the approximate extent of the caudad area.

process has been termed **receptive relaxation.** Because relaxation happens with each swallow, large volumes can be accommodated with a minimal rise in intragastric pressure. For example, the human stomach can accept 1600 cubic centimeters (cc) of air with a rise in pressure of no more than 10 mm Hg.

Receptive relaxation is mediated by a **vagovagal reflex,** a nervous reflex that has its afferent and efferent pathways in the vagus nerve. If this nerve is transected, receptive relaxation is impaired and the stomach becomes less distensible. Studies indicate that vagal impulses may act through 5-hydroxytryptamine receptors to release NO to cause the muscle to relax.

CLINICAL APPLICATIONS

Contractions of pharyngeal muscle are controlled solely by extrinsic nerves. Therefore certain neurologic diseases (e.g., cerebrovascular accident) can have an adverse effect on this phase of swallowing. Aspiration often occurs because contractions in the pharynx and upper esophageal sphincter (UES) are no longer coordinated. A similar clinical picture can be seen in diseases that affect striated muscle or the myoneural junction.

Diseases affecting the smooth muscle portion of the esophagus predictably cause abnormalities in peristalsis and in the tone of the lower esophageal sphincter (LES). In **achalasia,** for example, the LES often fails to relax completely with swallowing. This may be coupled with a loss of peristalsis in the esophageal body, a complete absence of contractions, or the appearance of simultaneous rather than sequential contractions, with resulting impaired transit.

Patients with this disorder have considerable difficulty swallowing, often aspirate retained esophageal content, and may become severely malnourished. This disorder has been attributed to abnormalities in the enteric nerves. In another disorder, **diffuse esophageal spasm,** simultaneous contractions of a long duration and high amplitude can occur. Affected persons have difficulty swallowing and may complain of chest pain. Although not always symptomatic, abnormalities in the esophageal component of swallowing can occur as part of a variety of systemic diseases. Examples are diabetes mellitus, chronic alcoholism, and scleroderma.

Motor dysfunction also can play an important contributory role in the pathogenesis of other esophageal diseases. The most common symptom associated with esophageal dysfunction is **heartburn.** This burning sensation is caused by the reflux of gastric acid into the esophagus and the resulting injury to the esophageal mucosa. This condition may be produced by motor abnormalities that result in abnormally low pressures in the LES or by the failure of secondary peristalsis to empty the esophagus effectively. Reflux may also

Continued

occur if intragastric pressure increases, as may occur following a large meal, during heavy lifting, or during pregnancy. Persistent reflux and the resulting inflammation lead to **gastroesophageal reflux disease** (GERD). This condition is usually treated effectively with inhibitors of gastric acid secretion. In some cases a region of the proximal stomach moves through the diaphragm into the thorax and produces severe gastric reflux. This condition is termed **hiatal hernia** and is often treated by surgery. Reflux itself is not abnormal, and it occurs several times a day. Under normal conditions the refluxed acid is cleared from the esophagus, and no symptoms develop.

Swallowing is assessed clinically by x-ray examination with barium and by esophageal manometry. In the x-ray study the patient swallows a bolus of liquid barium sulfate. Because this material is radiopaque, it can be observed fluoroscopically and recorded on the x-ray film as it traverses the esophagus, thereby providing a qualitative description of motor events in both the pharynx and the esophagus.

If a more detailed description of events is required or if motor disorders such as those just described are suspected, esophageal manometry is often useful. Catheters are passed through the nose or mouth so that their tips lie in various regions of the esophagus. Pressures detected by the catheters then are recorded between and during swallowing small sips of water. These recordings provide a quantitative description of events occurring in the sphincters and body of the esophagus.

A useful test for episodes of acid reflux is 24-hour monitoring of intraesophageal pH. A small pH probe is inserted nasally and positioned 5 cm above the lower esophageal sphincter. A small battery-powered computer is used for continuous recordings of pH.

SUMMARY

1. Swallowing is initiated voluntarily, but once initiated, it proceeds as an involuntary reflex.
2. Swallowing is accomplished by peristaltic contraction of pharyngeal muscles, during which time the UES relaxes. This is followed by peristaltic contraction of the esophageal musculature, during which time the LES and the orad region of the stomach relax.
3. Peristaltic contraction of the pharyngeal muscles, relaxation of the UES, and peristaltic contraction of the striated muscle of the upper esophagus are regulated by pathways within the central nervous system. Peristaltic contraction of the smooth muscle of the lower esophagus and relaxation of the LES are regulated by pathways within the central nervous system and by pathways within the intrinsic nerves.

4. Contraction of the pharynx and esophagus can be initiated by swallowing (primary peristalsis). Contraction of the esophagus can be initiated by stimulation of receptors within the esophagus (secondary peristalsis).
5. Tonic contraction of the LES between swallows is the result of an interplay of excitatory and inhibitory neural and hormonal influences acting on an intrinsic myogenic contraction. During a swallow, intrinsic nerves release a transmitter (perhaps NO or VIP) to cause muscle relaxation.
6. Contraction of the orad stomach is the result of an interplay of excitatory and inhibitory neural and hormonal influences acting on an intrinsic myogenic contraction. During a swallow, the orad stomach relaxes (receptive relaxation) in response to activation of inhibitory nerves in the vagus.

KEY WORDS AND CONCEPTS

Oral ingestion

Chewing reflex

Oropharynx

Tongue

Oral cavity

Nasopharynx

Glottis

Larynx

Peristaltic contraction

Pharynx

Upper esophageal sphincter

Swallowing center

Esophagus

Lower esophageal sphincter

Primary peristalsis

Secondary peristalsis

Vagotomy

Orad portion

Caudad portion

Receptive relaxation

Vasovagal reflex

Achalasia

Diffuse esophageal spasm

Heartburn

Gastroesophageal reflux disease

Hiatal hernia

SUGGESTED READINGS

Biancani P, Harnett KM, Behar J: Esophageal motor function. In Yamada T, Alpers DH, Laine L, et al: ed 3, *Textbook of Gastroenterology*, vol 1, Philadelphia, 1999, Lippincott Williams & Wilkins.

Mittal RK: Motor function of the pharynx, the esophagus, and its sphincters. In Johnson LR, editor: ed 5, *Physiology of the Gastrointestinal Tract*, vol 1, San Diego, 2012, Elsevier.

Roman C, Gonella J: Extrinsic control of digestive tract motility. In Johnson LR, editor: ed 2, *Physiology of the Gastrointestinal Tract*, vol 1, New York, 1987, Raven Press.

Shaker R: Pharyngeal motor function. In Johnson LR, editor: ed 4, *Physiology of the Gastrointestinal Tract*, vol 1, San Diego, 2006, Elsevier.

Tack J: Neurophysiologic mechanisms of gastric reservoir function. In Johnson LR, editor: ed 5, *Physiology of the Gastrointestinal Tract*, vol 1, San Diego, 2012, Elsevier.

4 GASTRIC EMPTYING

OBJECTIVES

- Describe the contractions of the orad and caudad regions of the stomach.
- Explain the regulation of the contractile activity of the stomach, including the role of slow waves.
- List the components of the gastric contents that affect the rate of gastric emptying.
- Understand the role of duodenal receptors in the regulation of gastric emptying.
- Describe the changes in motility that regulate gastric emptying.
- Describe the disorders that may result in an impairment of gastric emptying.

Motility of the stomach and upper small intestine is organized to accomplish the orderly emptying of contents into the duodenum in the presence of ingested material of variable quantity and composition. Accommodation and temporary storage of ingested material result from receptive relaxation of the orad stomach (see Chapter 3). Emptying, which also requires mixing ingested material with gastric juice and reducing the particle size of any solids that have been swallowed, results from integrated contractions of the orad stomach, caudad stomach, pylorus, and duodenum.

ANATOMIC CONSIDERATIONS

Gastric contractions result from activity of smooth muscle cells that are arranged in three layers: an outer longitudinal layer, a middle circular layer, and an inner oblique layer. The **longitudinal layer** is absent on the anterior and posterior surfaces of the stomach. The **circular layer** is the most prominent and is present in all areas of the stomach except the paraesophageal region. The **oblique layer,** the least complete, is formed from two bands of muscle lying on the anterior and posterior surfaces. These two bands meet at the gastroesophageal sphincter and fan out to fuse with the circular muscle layer in the caudad part of the stomach. Both the circular and the longitudinal muscle layers increase in thickness toward the duodenum.

The stomach is richly innervated with both intrinsic and extrinsic nerves. The intrinsic nerves lie in various plexuses, the most prominent being the myenteric plexus, which lies in a three-dimensional matrix between the longitudinal and circular muscle layers and throughout the circular muscle layer. The myenteric plexus receives nerve endings from other intrinsic plexuses, as well as from extrinsic nerves. Axons from neurons within the myenteric plexus synapse with the muscle fibers and with glandular cells of the stomach. Extrinsically the stomach is innervated by branches of the vagus nerves and by fibers originating in the celiac plexus of the sympathetic nervous system.

The **pylorus,** or gastroduodenal junction, is characterized by a thickening of the circular muscle layer of the distal antrum. Separating this bundle of muscle from the duodenum is a connective tissue septum; however, some of the longitudinal muscle fibers pass from the antrum to connect with muscle cells of the duodenum. The pylorus is richly innervated with both extrinsic and intrinsic nerves, and nerve endings within the thickened circular muscle layer are abundant. Many of these endings contain neuropeptides, especially enkephalin, and many produce and release nitric oxide (NO).

The anatomy of the proximal duodenum is similar to that of the rest of the intestine (described in Chapter 5). A significant difference is the larger number of intrinsic nerves present in this area compared with the rest of the small bowel. These nerves may be involved in the regulation of gastric emptying (described in a later section).

In addition to the muscle cells and nerves, interstitial cells of Cajal (ICCs) also are prominent in all regions and appear to play a prominent role in regulating motility. Many ICCs form gap junctions with smooth muscle cells, whereas others appear to create a bridge between nerve endings and smooth muscle cells.

CONTRACTIONS OF THE ORAD REGION OF THE STOMACH

As detailed in the previous chapter, the predominant motor activity of the orad region of the stomach is the accommodation of ingested material. The musculature of the orad stomach is thin, contractions are weak, and during the remainder of the digestive state, pressures are essentially equal to intra-abdominal pressure, with superimposed tonic pressure changes. These pressure changes are predominantly of low amplitude and have durations of 1 minute or more. The contractions that produce these pressure changes reduce the size of the stomach as the stomach empties. These tonic contractions result in accommodation of the remaining gastric contents and propulsion of those contents into the caudad stomach. A consequence of this minimal contractile activity is that little mixing of ingested contents occurs in the orad stomach. Contents often remain in relatively undisturbed layers for an hour or more after eating. As a result, salivary amylase (see Chapter 7), which is inactivated by gastric acid, can digest a significant portion of the starch present in a meal. Little is known about the regulation of contractions in the orad stomach during digestion. Both gastrin and cholecystokinin (CCK) decrease contractions and increase gastric distensibility. However, only the effect of CCK appears to be physiologic.

CONTRACTIONS OF THE CAUDAD REGION OF THE STOMACH

In the fasted state, the stomach is mostly quiescent. After eating, phasic contractions of variable intensity occur almost continuously. Contractions normally begin in the midstomach and move toward the gastroduodenal junction (Fig. 4-1). Thus the primary contractile event is a **peristaltic contraction.** As contractions approach the gastroduodenal junction, they increase in both force and velocity. At any one locus of the human stomach, the duration of each contraction ranges between 2 and 20 seconds, and the maximum frequency is approximately three contractions per minute. Between contractions, pressures in the caudad region are near intra-abdominal levels.

Contractions of the caudad region of the stomach serve to both mix and propel gastric contents. Once a contraction begins in the midportion of the stomach, gastric contents are propelled toward the gastroduodenal junction (Fig. 4-2, *A*). As the contraction approaches the gastroduodenal junction, some contents are evacuated into the duodenum (Fig. 4-2, *B*). However, because the peristaltic wave increases in velocity as it approaches the junction, the contraction overtakes the gastric contents. Once this occurs, most

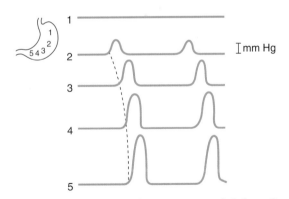

FIGURE 4-1 ■ Intraluminal pressures recorded from five areas of the stomach. A sensor in the orad region records little phasic activity. Sensors in the caudad region detect peristaltic contractions, which begin in the midportion of the stomach and progress toward the gastroduodenal junction. The contractions increase in force and velocity as they near the junction, and they repeat at multiple intervals of 12 to 20 seconds. The presence and force of contractions depend on the digestive state of the individual.

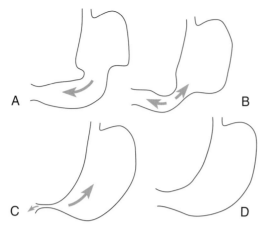

FIGURE 4-2 ■ Effects of gastric peristaltic contractions on intraluminal contents. **A,** The contraction begins in the midregion of the stomach and pushes contents toward the duodenum. **B,** As the contraction increases in force and velocity, some of the contents are passed over and are forced back into the body of the stomach. **C,** Contraction force and velocity are great enough to cause rapid and almost complete closure of the distal antrum. Before and during this contraction, a portion of the contents is propelled into the duodenum. However, most is propelled back into the body of the stomach. **D,** No gross movement of the gastric contents occurs between contractions.

of the contents are propelled back into the main body of the stomach (Fig. 4-2, *C*), where they remain until the next contraction sequence (Fig. 4-2, *D*). This propulsion back into the stomach has been termed **retropulsion.** Retropulsion causes a thorough mixing of the gastric contents and mechanically reduces the size of solid particles. (See videos: http://www.wzw.tum.de/humanbiology/motvid01/movie_11_1mot01.wmv; http://www.wzw.tum.de/humanbiology/motvid01/movie_13_1mot01.wmv; accessed March 2013).

Contractions of the caudad area of the stomach are controlled by interactions among smooth muscle cells and ICCs, as well as by nervous and humoral elements. Smooth muscle cells in this area have a membrane potential that fluctuates rhythmically with cyclic depolarizations and repolarizations. These fluctuations are called **slow waves** (also referred to as *basic electric rhythm, pacesetter potentials,* and *control activity*). Slow waves have two components: an initial upstroke potential and a secondary plateau potential. In the stomach, slow waves can initiate significant contractions; thus some investigators refer to them as *action potentials.* However, slow waves are always present,

regardless of the presence or absence of contractions. Their frequency is constant, and humans have approximately 3 cycles/minute (cpm). When slow waves are recorded from multiple sites between the midstomach and the gastroduodenal junction, they have the same frequency at all sites (Fig. 4-3). However, slow waves do not occur simultaneously at all points along the stomach. Rather, a phase lag occurs; thus, they seem to pass from an area in the midstomach toward the gastroduodenal junction. This phase lag between slow waves at equidistant points lessens as the gastroduodenal junction is neared. The frequency and velocity of the peristaltic waves are therefore controlled by the frequency and velocity of spread of the slow wave.

Nervous and humoral factors are not necessary for the presence of slow waves, but they do alter slow wave behavior. Vagotomy disorganizes the slow waves so that the phase lag varies in both duration and direction. The hormone gastrin increases the frequency of gastric slow waves, although it has little effect on the apparent propagation of the waves through the musculature.

Simultaneous recordings of both electrical and mechanical activities have shown that slow waves initiate significant contractions of the musculature only when the plateau potential exceeds a threshold (Fig. 4-4). Once the threshold is exceeded, the greater the amplitude of the plateau, the greater will be the force of contraction. The plateau potential may or may not be accompanied by superimposed rapid oscillations called **spike potentials** or **spike bursts.** These oscillations also appear to initiate contractions and are seen more frequently in muscle of the caudad antrum. Threshold values for contraction are not reached by every slow wave. Therefore not every slow wave is accompanied by a contraction. If the threshold is reached, it is only during a specific phase of the slow wave cycle. Thus the phasic and peristaltic nature of gastric contractions results from the presence of slow waves.

Whether an individual slow wave results in a contraction and the amplitude of contractions are determined by hormonal and neural activity, which in turn depends on the digestive state of the individual and the nature of the gastric contents. These events regulate not only the level of the plateau of the slow wave but also the amount of spiking and therefore both the frequency and strength of contractions. Vagal nerve transection leads to a decrease in contractions, whereas vagal

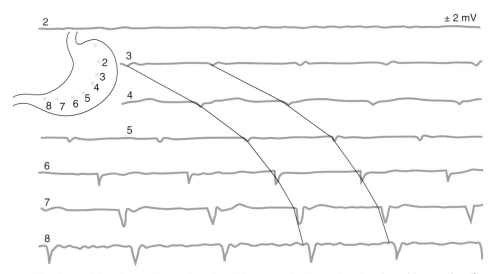

FIGURE 4-3 ▨ Electrical activity of smooth muscle cells of the stomach. Electrodes placed on the serosal surface record no changes from the orad region. In the midregion, however, slow waves occur continuously at intervals of 12 to 20 seconds. Slow waves give the appearance of moving through the caudad region at increasing velocities. Compare this with Figure 4-1. mV, microvolts. *(Adapted from Kelly KA, Code CF, Elveback LR: Patterns of canine gastric electrical activity. Am J Physiol 217:461-471, 1969.)*

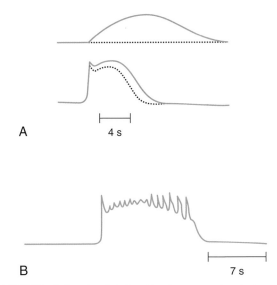

FIGURE 4-4 ▨ **A,** Relationship between electrical and mechanical activities of smooth muscle from the caudad region of the stomach. *Bottom tracing* depicts two slow waves (action potentials) superimposed. *Top tracing* depicts mechanical events associated with the potential changes. Note that a contraction is initiated only by the slow wave of larger amplitude and longer duration. **B,** Slow wave potential recorded from distal antrum. Note the oscillations and spike potentials during plateau. *(A, Adapted from Szurszewski JH: Mechanism of action of pentagastrin and acetylcholine on the longitudinal muscle of the canine antrum. J Physiol 252:335-361, 1975; B, Adapted from El-Sharkaway TY, Morgan KG, Szurszewski JH: Intracellular electrical activity of canine and human gastric smooth muscle. J Physiol 279:291-307, 1978.)*

stimulation increases the number and force of contractions. Usually, sympathetic nerve activity depresses contractions. Gastrin and motilin increase contractions, whereas secretin and gastric inhibitory peptide (GIP) inhibit them. The physiologic significance of the gastric motor effects of secretin and GIP is doubtful.

CONTRACTIONS OF THE GASTRODUODENAL JUNCTION

The question whether a true sphincter exists between the stomach and the duodenum is unsettled. There is a definite difference in the contractile activities of the stomach, on one side, and of the duodenum, on the other. One contracts at a frequency of approximately 3 cpm, and the other contracts at approximately 12 cpm. The thickened ring of circular muscle between the two organs appears to behave independently. In humans, some investigators have demonstrated a zone of elevated pressure between the stomach and the duodenum (an indication of sphincteric activity); other investigators, however, have not found such an area. Studies show that even if a zone of elevated pressure is not found, the pylorus can contract independently, thus altering the resistance to flow between the stomach and duodenum (Fig. 4-5). This action can have a large effect on gastric emptying.

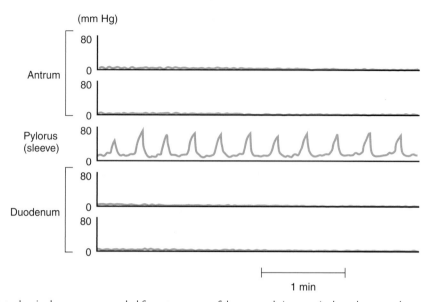

FIGURE 4-5 ■ Intraluminal pressures recorded from two areas of the stomach (antrum), the pylorus, and two areas of the proximal duodenum during the intraduodenal infusion of lipid. Note the regular isolated contractions, and the elevated pressures (0 indicates atmospheric pressure in each tracing) between contractions, in the pylorus. This activity is occurring at a time when no contractions are present in the stomach and duodenum. *(Adapted from Heddle R, Dent J, Read NW, et al: Antropyloroduodenal motor responses to intraduodenal lipid infusion in healthy volunteers. Am J Physiol 254:G671-G679, 1988.)*

CONTRACTIONS OF THE PROXIMAL DUODENUM

Duodenal contractions are mostly phasic. Although their maximum frequency can be approximately 12 per minute in the digestive state, these contractions seldom occur in a continuous manner. Rather, single, isolated contractions, or small groups of contractions, separated by intervals of no contractions, are the norm. In addition, duodenal contractions are not always peristaltic. Most contractions of the small intestine are of the segmenting type (see Chapter 5). Thus depending on their number and pattern, duodenal contractions either impede or facilitate the emptying of contents from the stomach.

REGULATION OF GASTRIC EMPTYING

Immediately after ingestion of a meal, the stomach may contain more than a liter of material, which takes several hours to leave the stomach and empty into the small intestine. Gastric emptying is accomplished by coordinated contractile activity of the stomach,

pylorus, and proximal small intestine (Fig. 4-6). Emptying appears to be regulated in a manner that allows for optimal intestinal digestion and absorption of foodstuffs (Fig. 4-7). Solids empty only after a lag period during which they are reduced in size by retropulsive activity of the caudad stomach. Only particles approximately 1 mm³ or smaller are readily emptied during the digestive phase of gastric motility. Conversely, liquids begin to empty almost immediately. The rate of emptying of both solids and liquids depends on their chemical compositions. Materials that are high in lipids or hydrogen (H^+) or that deviate markedly from isotonicity all empty at a slower rate than that observed for near-isotonic saline solutions.

Changes in gastric emptying are caused by alterations in the motility of the stomach, gastroduodenal junction, and duodenum. Decreases in distensibility of the orad stomach, increases in the force of peristaltic contractions of the caudad stomach, and increases in the diameter and inhibition of segmenting contractions of the proximal duodenum all lead to an increased rate of gastric emptying. Inhibition of emptying occurs

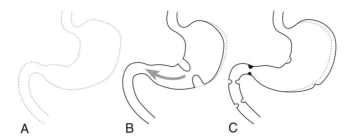

A   B   C

FIGURE 4-6 ■ Regulation of gastric emptying. **A,** Hypothetic conditions immediately after the rapid ingestion of a meal and before the onset of any contractile activity. This outline is superimposed in **B** and **C** to illustrate changes. **B,** Conditions favoring emptying are increased tone of the orad region of the stomach, forceful peristaltic contractions of the caudad region of the stomach, relaxation of the pylorus, and absence of segmenting contractions of the duodenum. As nutrients emptied from the stomach are further digested and absorbed in the small intestine, they excite receptors located in the intestinal mucosa. Activation of these receptors results in **C. C,** Relaxation of the orad region of the stomach, a decrease in the number and force of contractions of the caudad region of the stomach, contraction of the pylorus, and an increase in segmenting contractions of the duodenum. These actions result in a slowing of gastric emptying.

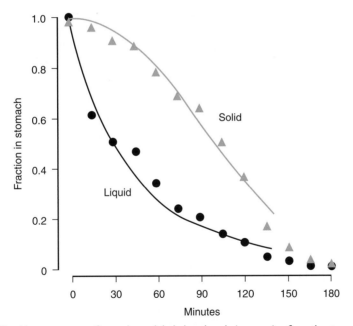

FIGURE 4-7 ■ Solid and liquid components of a meal were labeled so that their emptying from the stomach could be followed over time after ingestion of the meal. As indicated by the sharp decrease in the fraction remaining in the stomach, the liquid component began to empty almost immediately, and it also emptied more rapidly. Conversely, there was a lag time before the emptying of the label attached to the solid component, and this label emptied more slowly. The reason for this slower emptying was that the solid component had to be reduced to small particles before being emptied into the duodenum. *(Adapted from Camilleri M, Malagelada JR, Brown ML, et al: Relation between antral motility and gastric emptying of solids and liquids in humans. Am J Physiol 249:G580-G585, 1985.)*

on reversal of one or more of these contractile activities (see Fig. 4-6).

Regulation of emptying results from the presence of receptors that lie in the upper small bowel. These receptors respond to the physical properties (e.g., osmotic pressure) and chemical composition (e.g., H^+, lipids) of the intestinal contents. As contents empty from the stomach, **intestinal receptors** located in the duodenum are activated. Receptor activation triggers several neural and hormonal mechanisms that inhibit gastric emptying. For example, fats release CCK, which increases the distensibility of the orad stomach. Acid, when placed in the duodenum, inhibits motility and emptying with a latent period as short as 20 to 40 seconds, a finding indicating that the inhibition is the result of neural reflex. This reflex appears to be entirely intrinsic, with information from the duodenal receptors to the gastric smooth muscle carried by neurons of the intramural plexus. Other hormones such as secretin and GIP also inhibit emptying but do not appear to do so in physiologic concentrations. Neural input that activates the sympathetic system, such as that produced by pain, anxiety, fear, or even exercise, may slow gastric emptying. Much of the regulation of gastric emptying is mediated by as yet undefined pathways, but it is obvious that regulation allows time for osmotic equilibration, acid neutralization, and solubilization and digestion of lipids.

The pattern of motility of the gastroduodenal area changes after the nutrient components of the meal have been digested and absorbed. Any large particles of undigested residue that remain in the stomach are emptied by a burst of peristaltic contractions (phase 3) as part of the migrating motor complex (MMC) (Fig. 4-8). During this short burst, powerful contractions begin in the previously inactive orad region and sweep the entire length of the stomach. The pylorus dilates and the duodenum relaxes during each sweep so that the resistance to emptying is minimal. Then **duodenal contractions** sweep the contents onward (see Chapter 5). (See video: http://www.wzw.tum.de/humanbiology /motvid02/movie_06_1mot02.wmv; accessed March 2013). After a burst of activity, the region remains relaxed for an hour or more. Then intermittent contractions begin and lead to another burst. This cycle repeats every 90 minutes or so until ingestion of the next meal. Premature bursts can be initiated by injection of the hormone motilin and by drugs (e.g., erythromycin) thought to act on motilin receptors.

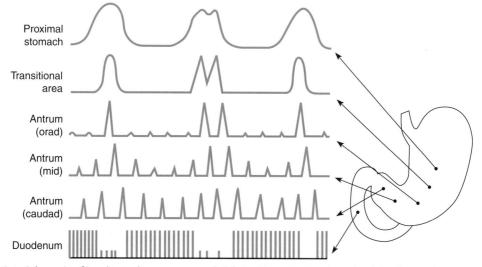

FIGURE 4-8 ▨ Schematic of intraluminal pressures recorded from the stomach and proximal duodenum during an active phase of a migrating motor complex. Phasic contractions begin in the orad region of the stomach and propagate over the caudad region. As contractions of the caudad region approach the gastroduodenal junction, the pylorus relaxes *(not shown)* and duodenal contractions are momentarily inhibited. This process allows contents to be swept into the duodenum. Contents are then propelled toward the colon, as described in Chapter 5. *(Adapted from Malagelada JR, Azpiroz F: Determinants of gastric emptying and transit in the small intestine. In Schultz SG, Wood JD, Rauner BB [eds]: The Gastrointestinal System, vol 1. Bethesda, MD, American Physiological Society, 1989.)*

CLINICAL APPLICATIONS

Disorders of gastric motility generally are manifested by a rate of gastric emptying that is either too slow or too fast. This condition may reflect an abnormality in one or all of the major motor functions of the stomach. When the stomach fails to empty properly, the affected person experiences nausea, loss of appetite, and early satiety, and gastric contents often may be vomited. The most common cause of impaired emptying is obstruction at the gastric outlet. Examples of disorders that may result in obstruction are gastric cancer and peptic ulcer disease. In the latter, the gastric lumen at the pylorus may actually become occluded from inflammation and scarring associated with the ulcer. Impaired emptying also can be caused by the absence or disorganization of motor events in the caudad stomach. These phenomena occur with a variety of metabolic disorders, such as diabetes mellitus and potassium depletion.

Vagus nerve section **(vagotomy)** invariably leads to a delay in gastric emptying of solids. Consequently, vagotomy (e.g., performed to decrease acid secretion in peptic ulcer disease) is coupled with surgical alterations of the pylorus **(pyloroplasty)** or creation of a new gastric outlet **(gastroenterostomy)** in an attempt to avoid this complication. After such an operation, emptying of liquids generally is accelerated, but even with alteration of the gastric outlet, emptying of solids still may be slowed. Most patients undergoing this type of surgical procedure experience no other symptoms. However, some may experience diarrhea, sweating, palpitations, cramps, and a variety of other unpleasant symptoms, which may be the result of rapid emptying that constitutes **dumping syndrome.** This in turn causes the rapid entry of large volumes of fluid into the upper small bowel to bring the hypertonic contents to isotonicity.

It is speculated that motility abnormalities may underlie or contribute to other diseases of the upper gastrointestinal tract. For example, gastric emptying is accelerated in patients with a duodenal ulcer. This accelerated emptying may enhance the delivery of gastric acid to the duodenum and perhaps may overwhelm the ability of the duodenal mucosa to defend itself against injury. Alternatively, for patients with a gastric ulcer, gastric emptying appears to be slowed. This slowing may render the stomach more susceptible to injury.

CLINICAL TESTS

A qualitative assessment of gastric motility and emptying can be obtained by x-ray and fluoroscopic evaluation of a barium-filled stomach. Aspiration of the stomach at specific intervals after instillation of an isotonic saline solution also gives information on gastric emptying. A more quantitative test involves gamma scintigraphy. For this test, radiolabeled liquid or solid food, or both, is ingested, and gamma cameras are used to scan the stomach at various times afterward. The fraction of material remaining in the stomach is then plotted as a function of time (see Fig. 4-7). In certain laboratories, manometry similar to that used in assessing esophageal motility can be employed. Compliance of the orad stomach can be assessed using a "barostat," a large bag placed in the stomach that monitors changes in volume under set pressures. More recently, magnetic resonance imaging and ultrasonography have been employed as noninvasive methods to assess gastric motility and emptying.

SUMMARY

1. Contractile activity of the orad stomach varies with the digestive state. After the orad region has accommodated a meal, it exhibits low-amplitude, long-lasting contractions as the meal empties. After the meal has been digested and absorbed, the orad stomach undergoes periodic bursts of high-amplitude contractions as part of the MMC.

2. Contractions of the caudad stomach are mostly peristaltic, beginning in the midstomach and progressing toward the duodenum. During emptying of a meal, contractions are of variable amplitude and are more or less continuous at a frequency of approximately 3 cpm. During the interdigestive period, forceful peristaltic contractions are grouped into periodic bursts as part of the MMC.

3. Gastric emptying is highly regulated and involves feedback inhibition from receptors located in the upper small intestine. Receptors are stimulated by osmotic pressure, H^+, and fatty acids. Stimulation results in patterns of motility that slow emptying: decreased tonic contraction of the orad stomach, decreased force and number of contractions of the caudad stomach, increased tone and phasic contractions of the pylorus, and increased segmenting contractions of the upper duodenum.

4. Rhythmic membrane depolarizations and repolarizations called slow waves occur in smooth muscle cells of the caudad stomach. These waves are omnipresent, occurring at a frequency of approximately three per minute. Each depolarization appears to be initiated first in the midstomach and then to propagate toward the pylorus. Slow waves appear to set the timing and the peristaltic nature of contractions; however, not every slow wave initiates a contraction. Those that do are of large amplitude and may exhibit superimposed spike potentials.

5. Vagotomy results in a decrease in the number and force of contractions of the caudad stomach and a decrease in gastric emptying of solids. Motilin induces contractions that are part of the gastric phase of the MMC.

KEY WORDS AND CONCEPTS

Longitudinal layer	Intestinal receptors
Circular layer	Duodenal contractions
Oblique layer	Vagotomy
Pylorus	Pyloroplasty
Peristaltic contraction	Gastroenterostomy
Retropulsion	Dumping syndrome
Slow waves	
Spike potentials/spike bursts	

SUGGESTED READINGS

Ehrlein HJ, Akkermans LMA: Gastric emptying. In Akkermans LMA, Johnson AG, Read NW, editors: *Gastric and Gastroduodenal Motility*, New York, 1984, Praeger.

Hasler WL: The physiology of gastric motility and gastric emptying. In Yamada T, Alpers DH, Laine L, et al: ed 3, *Textbook of Gastroenterology*, vol 1, Philadelphia, 1999, Lippincott Williams & Wilkins.

Hunt JN, Knox MT: Regulation of gastric emptying. In Code CF, editor: *Handbook of Physiology*, vol 4, Baltimore, 1968, Williams & Wilkins.

Rayner CK, Hebbard GS, Horowitz M: Physiology of the antral pump and gastric emptying. In Johnson LR, editor: ed 5, *Physiology of the Gastrointestinal Tract*, vol 1, San Diego, 2012, Elsevier.

5

MOTILITY OF THE SMALL INTESTINE

OBJECTIVES

- Compare the motility patterns of the small intestine during feeding and fasting.
- Describe the functions of slow waves and spike potentials in regulating contractions of the small intestine.
- Describe the functions and control of the migrating motility complex.
- Explain the peristaltic reflex and the intestino-intestinal reflex.
- Describe the motility changes that result in vomiting, and discuss the primary factors controlling it.

Motility of the small intestine is organized to optimize the processes of digestion and absorption of nutrients and the aboral propulsion of undigested material. Thus contractions perform at least three functions: (1) mixing of ingested foodstuffs with digestive secretions and enzymes, (2) circulation of all intestinal contents to facilitate contact with the intestinal mucosa, and (3) net propulsion of the intestinal contents in an aboral direction.

ANATOMIC CONSIDERATIONS

Contractions of the small intestine are effected by the activities of two layers of smooth muscle cells: an outer layer with the long axis of the cells arranged longitudinally and an inner layer with the long axis of the cells arranged circularly. In general, the circular muscle layer is thicker, and both layers are more abundant in the proximal intestine; they decrease in thickness distally to the level of the ileocecal junction.

The small intestine is richly innervated by elements of the autonomic nervous system. Within the wall of the intestine itself lie neurons, nerve endings, and receptors of the enteric nervous system. These neural elements tend to be concentrated in several plexuses. The most prominent, the **myenteric** or **Auerbach plexus,** lies between the circular and longitudinal layers of smooth muscle cells. Plexal neurons receive input from other neurons within the plexus, from receptors located in the mucosa and muscle walls, and from the central nervous system by way of the parasympathetic and sympathetic nerve trunks. Plexal neurons provide integrated output to smooth muscle cells of both muscle layers, to epithelial cells, and perhaps to endocrine and immune cells. Many neurotransmitters are present in the enteric nervous system, including acetylcholine, norepinephrine, vasoactive intestinal peptide, enkephalin, and other peptides. Furthermore, many nerves express nitric oxide synthase activity.

Interstitial cells of Cajal (ICCs) also are prominent in and adjacent to the enteric nerves and muscular layers of the intestine. At least two major classes of ICCs have been identified: those responsible for generating slow waves and those involved in mediating neural input to the smooth muscle cells.

Extrinsic innervation is supplied by the vagus nerve and by nerve fibers from the celiac and superior mesenteric ganglia (see Fig. 2-1). Many of the fibers within the vagus are preganglionic, whereas many from the abdominal ganglia are postganglionic. Some of the fibers within the vagus are cholinergic, whereas some from the abdominal plexuses are adrenergic. In addition, nerves that contain somatostatin, substance P, cholecystokinin (CCK), enkephalin, neuropeptide Y, and other transmitters have been identified in afferent and efferent vagal and splanchnic nerves. The exact pathways and physiologic roles of these nerves are being elucidated.

TYPES OF CONTRACTIONS

Between contractions, pressures within the lumen of the small intestine approximately equal the intra-abdominal pressure. When the musculature contracts, the lumen is occluded partially or totally, and the pressure increases. Most contractions are local events and involve only 1 to 4 centimeters (cm) of bowel at a time. The contractions usually produce intraluminal pressure waves that appear as nearly symmetric peaks of uniform shape (Fig. 5-1). In the human upper small bowel, contractions occur at any one site at multiple intervals of 5 seconds (Fig. 5-2).

Occasionally other types of pressure waves can be recorded. One such type consists of an elevated baseline pressure that lasts from 10 seconds to 8 minutes. This wave seldom occurs alone and is usually accompanied by superimposed phasic changes in pressure.

The effect of any contraction on the intestinal contents depends on the state of the musculature above and below the point of the contraction. If a contraction is not coordinated with activity above and below, intestinal contents are displaced both proximally and distally during the contraction and may flow back during the period of relaxation. This serves to mix and locally circulate the contents (Fig. 5-3, *A*). Such contractions appear to divide the bowel into segments, and this feature accounts for the name given to this process—**segmentation.** If, however, the contractions at adjacent sites occur in a proximal-to-distal sequence, aboral propulsion will result. (See video: http://www.wzw.tum.de/humanbiology/motvid01/movie_65_1mot01.wmv; accessed March 2013).

The small intestine is also capable of eliciting a highly coordinated contractile response that is propulsive in function. When an area of bowel is stimulated (e.g., by placement of a solid bolus of material in the lumen), the bowel responds with contraction orad and relaxation aboral to the point of stimulation. These events tend to move the material in an aboral direction (Fig. 5-3, *B*), and if they occur sequentially they can propel a bolus the entire length of the gut in a short time. This peristaltic response,

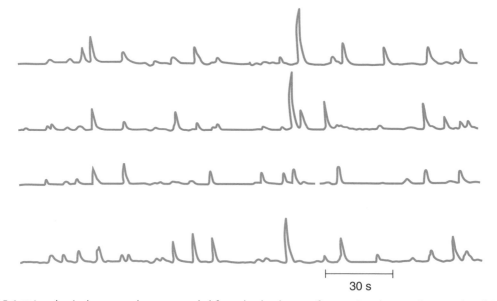

30 s

FIGURE 5-1 ■ Intraluminal pressure changes recorded from the duodenum of a conscious human. Sensors placed 1 cm apart record changes in pressure that are phasic, lasting 4 to 5 seconds. Note that a rather large contraction can take place at one site while nothing is recorded 1 cm away on either side.

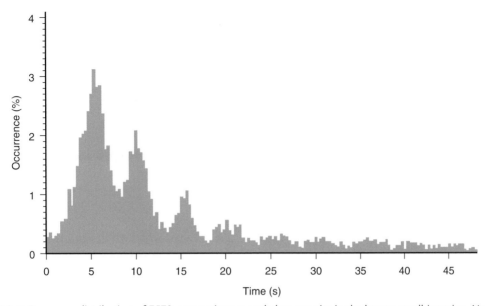

FIGURE 5-2 ■ Frequency distribution of 7572 contractions recorded at one site in the human small intestine. Note that the contractions are most frequent at multiples of 5 seconds, the approximate interval between slow waves in this region. *(From Christensen J, Glover JR., Macagno EO, et al: Statistics of contractions at a point in the human duodenum. Am J Physiol 221:1818-1823, 1971.)*

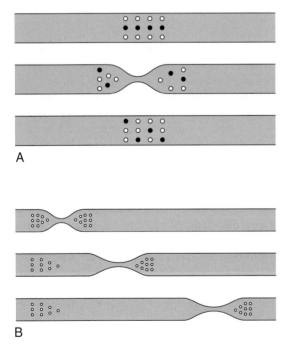

FIGURE 5-3 ■ The influence of contractions on contents within a region of intestine. Each panel depicts the region at three consecutive points in time. **A,** A contraction that is neither preceded nor followed by other contractions serves to mix and locally circulate the intestinal contents. **B,** Contractions that have an orad-to-caudad (left-to-right) sequence serve to propel contents in a net aboral direction.

first described by Bayliss and Starling, is known as the **law of the intestines.** Often it is invoked to explain how material is normally propelled through the small bowel. However, peristalsis involving long segments of intestine is seldom seen in normal persons, although peristaltic contractions involving short segments (1 to 4 cm) of intestine have been described.

PATTERNS OF CONTRACTIONS

Not only are there differences in individual contractions of the intestine, but there also are different patterns of contractions. In fasting humans, contractions do not occur evenly over time. Rather, at each locus cycles consisting of phases of no or few contractions are followed by a phase of intense contractions (phase 3) that ends abruptly (Fig. 5-4). The duration of each cycle is the same at adjacent loci of the bowel; however, the 5- to 10-minute phase of intense contractions does not occur simultaneously at all loci. Instead, this phase appears to migrate aborally, and it takes approximately 1.5 hours to sweep from the duodenum through the ileum. The characteristics of this pattern have earned it the title of **migrating motor complex** (MMC). This complex actually begins in the stomach (see Chapter 4).

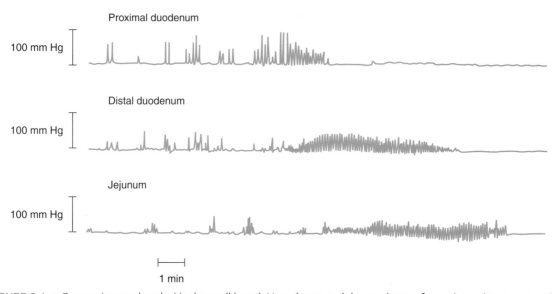

FIGURE 5-4 ■ Contractions at three loci in the small bowel. Note that at each locus, phases of no or intermittent contractions are followed by a phase of continuous contractions that ends abruptly. Also note that the phase of continuous contractions appears to migrate aborally along the bowel. Such a pattern is called the *migrating motor complex. (From Rees WD, Malagelada JR, Miller H: Human interdigestive and postprandial gastrointestinal motor and gastrointestinal hormone patterns. Dig Dis Sci 27:321-329, 1982.)*

(See videos: http://www.wzw.tum.de/humanbiology/ motvid02/movie_06_1mot02.wmv; http://www.wzw .tum.de/humanbiology/motvid02/movie_08_1mot02 .wmv; accessed March 2013). Its functions appear to be to sweep undigested contents from the stomach, through the small intestine, and into the colon and to maintain low bacterial counts in the upper intestine. MMCs cycle at intervals of approximately every 1.5 hours (Fig. 5-5) as long as the person is fasting.

In nonfasting persons, the MMC disappears, and contractions are spread more uniformly over time. In the human upper small bowel, contractions at any one site are present 14% to 34% of the recorded time. The most common pattern consists of one to three sequential contractions separated by periods of 5, 10, 15, or 20 seconds. These contractions are of variable intensity, with none as forceful as the intense contractions that occur during the MMC.

Contractions of the intestine are controlled by activities of the ICCs and smooth muscle cells, as well as by nerves and humoral substances. As in the stomach, smooth muscle cells in the small intestine have a membrane potential that fluctuates rhythmically with cyclic depolarizations and repolarizations of

5 to 15 millivolts (mV) (Fig. 5-6). This **slow wave activity** (or basic electrical rhythm) is always present whether contractions are occurring or not. At any one site in the intestine, slow wave frequency is constant. Frequency, however, is not the same at all levels of the bowel. There is a decrease in frequency toward the ileocecal junction. In humans the frequency decreases from a mean of approximately 12 cycles/minute (cpm) in the duodenum to a mean of approximately 8 cpm in the terminal ileum. The decrease is not linear because frequency is constant throughout the duodenum and for approximately 10 cm into the jejunum. Beyond that point, frequency declines more or less linearly.

Although slow wave frequency is the same over the proximal small intestine, slow waves do not occur simultaneously at all points. Multiple electrodes detect a proximal-to-distal phase lag that simulates a propagated signal (see Fig. 5-6).

Unlike in the stomach, slow waves themselves do not initiate contractions in the small intestine. Contractions are initiated by a second electrical event, often referred to as *spike potential activity*. **Spike potentials** are rapid depolarizations of the smooth muscle cell membrane that occur only during the

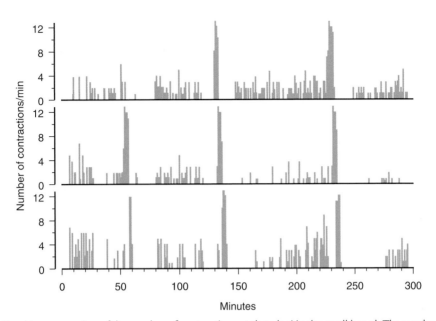

FIGURE 5-5 ■ Graphic presentation of the number of contractions at three loci in the small bowel. The number of contractions during each minute of the recording was counted and plotted against the time of recording. The resulting histogram indicates cycles of activity at each locus. Note that migrating motor complexes recur at each locus at intervals of approximately 100 minutes and that the phases of intense contractions appear to migrate aborally. *(From Vantrappen G, Janssens J: The interdigestive motor complex of normal subjects and patients with bacterial overgrowth of the small intestine. J Clin Invest 59:1158-1166, 1977.)*

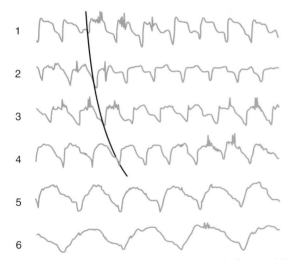

FIGURE 5-6 ■ Slow waves and spike potentials from multiple sites in the small intestine. Tracings 1 to 6 illustrate activity from progressively distal areas. The *solid line* connecting the slow waves in tracings 1 to 4 denotes the apparent propagation in the region of a slow wave frequency plateau. Tracings 5 and 6 show decreases in slow wave frequency at more distal areas. The rapid transients that occur on the peaks of some of the slow waves represent spike potentials.

depolarization phase of the slow wave. Because spike potentials are restricted to only one phase of the slow wave cycle, the contractions they initiate are phasic. The muscle relaxes during the repolarization phase of the slow wave cycle.

During periods when every slow wave is accompanied by spike potentials, the intestine at any site contracts at the same frequency as the slow wave frequency at that site. Thus slow wave frequency sets the maximum frequency of contractions at any one site. In addition, because a gradient exists in the slow wave frequency along the small bowel, there is a gradient in the maximal frequency of contractions. For most of the time, however, spike potentials do not accompany every slow wave. During these periods, contractions at any one site occur at multiples of the slow wave interval. Thus it is no coincidence that in the human proximal bowel, slow waves occur every 5 seconds and contractions occur at multiple intervals of 5 seconds.

Although slow waves at adjacent sites along the bowel are always present and are temporally related, the occurrence of spike potentials is often localized. Thus sites 1 to 2 cm on either side of an area exhibiting slow waves with spike potentials may exhibit slow waves only. When this is the situation, segmenting contractions occur. Conversely, when the occurrence of spike potentials is not localized, slow waves do influence the spatial relationships of contractions at adjacent sites. The phase lag in occurrence of slow waves at adjacent sites imposes a phase lag in the occurrence of contractions at adjacent sites.

As explained previously, not every slow wave is accompanied by spike potentials and muscle contraction. The occurrence of spike potentials and contractions is regulated by nervous activity and by circulating and locally released chemical agents. Certain reflexes depend on the intrinsic neurons, the extrinsic neurons, or both. The **peristaltic reflex** (law of the intestines) described previously depends on an intact enteric nervous system. Application of neural blocking agents abolishes or greatly reduces this reflex. Another reflex, the **intestino-intestinal reflex,** depends on extrinsic neural connections. If an area of the bowel is grossly distended, contractile activity in the rest of the bowel is inhibited. Sectioning of the extrinsic nerves abolishes this reflex. Additionally, it is well known that changes in emotional state can induce alterations in small bowel motility. Thus the small bowel is under the influence of higher centers of the nervous system.

In addition to neural control, many circulating and endogenously released chemicals alter intestinal motility. Epinephrine released from the adrenal glands tends to inhibit contractions. Serotonin, which is contained in large quantities within the small intestine, stimulates contractions, as do certain of the prostaglandins.

Several hormones also alter intestinal motility. Gastrin, CCK, motilin, and insulin tend to stimulate contractions, whereas secretin and glucagon tend to inhibit them. The exact role of these chemical agents in the regulation of motility is yet to be clarified.

The presence of a characteristic pattern of contractions during fasting—the MMC—indicates complex controlling mechanisms. The hormone motilin may be involved in regulating MMC cycle length. Plasma levels of motilin fluctuate with the same periodicity as for the phase of intense duodenal contractions, and exogenously administered motilin initiates a premature MMC. Enteric nerves also are involved because their disruption alters MMC initiation and migration. Extrinsic nerves do not seem to be required. Segments of intestine that have been extrinsically denervated still exhibit MMCs. However, extrinsic neural activity can modify characteristics of the MMC.

Feeding abolishes MMCs and institutes a pattern of more or less continuous contractions of varying amplitude. The change in pattern caused by feeding probably is brought about by hormones such as gastrin and CCK, which are released during feeding, and by neural mechanisms.

VOMITING

Vomiting (emesis) is the forceful expulsion of intestinal and gastric contents through the mouth. General discharge of the autonomic nervous system precedes and accompanies vomiting, with resulting copious salivation, sweating, rapid breathing, and an irregular heartbeat. In humans vomiting is usually, but not necessarily, associated with the feeling of nausea. Vomiting is normally preceded by retching, which is the pattern of activity that overcomes the antireflux mechanisms of the gastrointestinal (GI) tract.

A wave of reverse peristalsis beginning in the distal small intestine moves intestinal contents orad. Retching begins as this wave moves through the duodenum. A retch begins with a deep inspiration against a closed glottis and a strong contraction of the abdominal muscles. This increases intra-abdominal pressure and decreases intrathoracic pressure, so that the pressure gradient between these portions of the GI tract may become as great as 200 mm Hg. With each retch, the abdominal portion of the esophagus and a portion of the stomach actually slide through the hiatus of the diaphragm and move into the thorax. A contraction of the antrum and continued reverse peristalsis force the gastric contents through a relaxed lower esophageal sphincter and into the flaccid esophagus. As the retch subsides, the stomach moves back into the relaxed abdomen, and most of the contents drain back into the stomach. The cycle may be repeated several times, during which the upper esophageal sphincter remains closed, thus preventing gastric contents from entering the pharynx or mouth.

Vomiting itself occurs after a sequence of stronger or developed retches. A sudden strong contraction of the abdominal muscles raises the diaphragm high into the thorax and results in an increase in intrathoracic pressure that may equal 100 mm Hg. The larynx and hyoid bone are then reflexively drawn forward, and the increased intrathoracic pressure forces the contents of the esophagus past the upper esophageal sphincter and out of the mouth. Material remaining in the esophagus empties into the stomach after the abdominal muscles relax. The cycle may be repeated until almost all the contents have been expelled.

Vomiting can be induced by a variety of diverse stimuli, both peripheral and central in origin. These include pain, foul odors, repulsive sights, and psychological factors acting at the level of the cerebral cortex. A group of receptors located in the floor of the fourth ventricle of the brain, which is outside the blood-brain barrier, constitutes a chemoreceptor trigger zone that is activated by emetics in the blood or cerebrospinal fluid. Stimulation of this zone also occurs during motion sickness caused by unequal vestibular input. In addition, chemically responsive receptors occur in the GI tract and respond to emetics such as ipecac. Vomiting is also triggered by mechanical stimuli to the GI tract, such as induced by tickling the back of the throat and by distention or blockage of the stomach or intestines. All these stimuli converge on neurons located in the medulla, which interact with additional medullary neurons controlling retching. Electrical stimulation of neurons in these areas can cause vomiting without retching or retching without vomiting. In the normal situation, however, their activities are closely coordinated.

In general, vomiting is a protective mechanism to rid the body of noxious or toxic substances. Prolonged vomiting, however, can cause severe problems in fluid and electrolyte balance, especially in children. Because gastric juice contains relatively (to plasma) high concentrations of hydrogen (H^+) and potassium (K^+), these individuals may develop metabolic alkalosis and hypokalemia.

CLINICAL APPLICATIONS

Primary disorders of small intestine motility are rare. The small intestine may be involved in certain general disorders of smooth muscle of the gastrointestinal and urinary tracts. The cause of these disorders is unknown, but they may have a genetic basis in some patients. When the disorder is clinically apparent, a patient will appear to have episodes of intestinal obstruction; however, the problem seems to involve a failure of propulsive motility rather than an obstruction. Thus the name **idiopathic pseudo-obstruction** has been coined. In some patients with this syndrome, the smooth muscle cells and interstitial cells of Cajal are involved. In other patients, histologic studies show changes in enteric nerves.

Altered small intestinal motility resulting in delayed transit frequently accompanies a variety of diseases and clinical conditions. Perhaps the most common is the transient ileus or apparent paralysis of the small intestine sometimes seen after abdominal surgery. However, intra-abdominal inflammation (e.g., pancreatitis, appendicitis, abscess) may produce a similar picture. Systemic diseases such as diabetes mellitus and amyloidosis, metabolic alterations such as potassium depletion, and administration of drugs, particularly anticholinergics, all may have an adverse effect on intestinal transit. Mixing probably is impaired as well, although this is less clinically apparent.

Alternatively, rapid intestinal transit is seen in certain malabsorptive states induced by infectious agents, allergic reaction, and various pharmacologic agents. In these conditions both motility and absorption are affected. In most disease states it is not clear whether changes in motility are primary (caused by the disease) or secondary (caused by the presence of unabsorbed or secreted material).

CLINICAL TESTS

Auscultation to detect "bowel sounds" probably is the most common means used to assess bowel activity. In addition, observing the movement of barium by x-ray studies and of isotopes by scintigraphy (see Chapter 4) can yield some information on transit time through the small bowel. Unfortunately, these methods are not precise. Advances in technology have made the recording of intraluminal pressures rather easy in normal persons and in patients with minimal gastrointestinal dysfunction. However, the inaccessibility of the small intestine and the difficulty in placing intraluminal sensors in patients with major dysmotility limit the routine use of direct recordings of intestinal contractions as a diagnostic tool.

SUMMARY

1. Movement of contents within the intestinal lumen depends on the type of contraction. Segmenting contractions cause mixing and local circulation of contents. Peristaltic contractions cause net aboral transit.

2. During digestion of a meal, most contractions are of the segmenting type, with short peristaltic contractions occurring randomly. During interdigestive periods, bursts of intense peristaltic contractions envelop each region of the intestine approximately every 90 minutes. Each burst appears to begin in the stomach and migrate aborally along the intestine such that it reaches the terminal ileum in approximately 90 minutes. This activity is called the MMC.

3. Intestinal slow waves are cyclic depolarizations and repolarizations of muscle cell membranes. At any locus of the intestine, slow waves are present at a constant frequency (i.e., approximately 12 cpm in the duodenum and 8 cpm in the ileum). At adjacent loci, slow waves appear to propagate aborally.

4. Spike potentials are rapid fluctuations in membrane potential that are superimposed on the depolarization phase of the slow wave. These potentials, not the slow waves themselves, initiate contractions of the muscle. Spike potentials do not accompany every slow wave. Their presence and pattern depend on the digestive state and on neural and humoral activities.

5. Enteric nerves coordinate both the types and patterns of contractions. The phase of intense contractions of the MMC in the upper intestine may be initiated by the release of motilin. The conversion of the MMC pattern to the digestive pattern may result in part from the release of hormones such as gastrin and CCK.

6. Vomiting in humans usually involves nausea and retching, which overcomes the antireflux mechanisms of the GI tract, and occurs in response to a variety of stimuli that are coordinated in the medulla.

KEY WORDS AND CONCEPTS

Myenteric/Auerbach plexus

Segmentation

Law of the intestines

Migrating motor complex

Slow wave activity

Spike potentials

Peristaltic reflex

Intestino-intestinal reflex

Idiopathic pseudo-obstruction

SUGGESTED READINGS

Hasler WL: Small intestinal motility. In Johnson LR, editor: ed 4, *Physiology of the Gastrointestinal Tract*, vol 1, San Diego, 2006, Elsevier.

Weisbrodt NW: Motility of the small intestine. In Johnson LR, editor: ed 2, *Physiology of the Gastrointestinal Tract*, vol 1, New York, 1987, Raven Press.

Wingate DL: Backward and forward with the migrating complex, *Dig Dis Sci* 26:641–666, 1981.

MOTILITY OF THE LARGE INTESTINE

OBJECTIVES

- Describe the anatomy of the large intestine.
- Explain the function of the ileocecal reflex.
- Define a mass movement.
- Understand the motility of defecation and the rectosphincteric reflex.
- Discuss the control of defecation and explain the loss of control that occurs with some spinal cord injuries.

Contractions of the large intestine are organized to allow for optimal absorption of water and electrolytes, net aboral movement of contents, and storage and orderly evacuation of feces.

ANATOMIC CONSIDERATIONS

Anatomically the human large intestine is divided into the following: the **cecum**; the **ascending, transverse, descending,** and **sigmoid colon**; the **rectum**; and the **anal canal.** The muscular layers of the large intestine are composed of both longitudinally and circularly arranged fibers. Longitudinal fibers are concentrated into three flat bands called the **taeniae coli.** These run from the cecum to the rectum, where the fibers fan out to form a more continuous longitudinal coat. The circular layer of muscle fibers is continuous from the cecum to the anal canal, where it increases in thickness to form the **internal anal sphincter.** Overlapping and slightly distal to the internal anal sphincter are layers of striated muscle. These striated muscle bundles make up the **external anal sphincter.**

In humans the external features of the large intestine differ from those of the small intestine. In addition to the presence of taeniae coli, the colon appears to be divided into segments called **haustra** or **haustrations** (Fig. 6-1). Haustra probably are the result of structural and functional properties of the colon. Points of concentration of muscular tissue and mucosal foldings can be found in colons examined post mortem.

In addition, haustra are more prominent in areas of the colon that possess taeniae coli. Haustra are not fixed, however. Segmental colonic contractions appear, disappear, and form again at another locus. Thus haustral formation also has a dynamic component because of the contractile activity of colonic musculature.

The large intestine, like other areas of the bowel, is innervated by the autonomic nervous system (ANS). The enteric system consists partly of many nerve cell bodies and endings that lie between the circular and the longitudinal muscle coats. In areas of the large intestine with taeniae, this myenteric plexus is concentrated beneath them. Cells of the myenteric plexus receive input from a variety of receptors within the intestine, as well as by way of the extrinsic nerves. Axons from these cells innervate the muscle layers. Extrinsic innervation to the large intestine comes from both parasympathetic and sympathetic branches of the ANS. There are two pathways of parasympathetic innervation: the cecum and the ascending and transverse portions of the colon are innervated by the vagus nerve; the descending and sigmoid areas of the colon and the rectum are innervated by pelvic nerves from the sacral region of the spinal cord. The pelvic nerves enter the colon near the rectosigmoid junction and project orally and aborally within the plane of the myenteric plexus. These projections, called **shunt fascicles,** innervate myenteric nerves en route. The vagus and pelvic nerves consist primarily of preganglionic efferent fibers and many afferent fibers. The efferent fibers synapse with the nerve cell bodies of the myenteric and other intrinsic plexuses. The proximal regions of the large intestine are sympathetically innervated by fibers that originate from the superior mesenteric ganglion. More distal regions receive input from the inferior mesenteric ganglion. The distal rectum and anal canal are innervated by sympathetic fibers

from the hypogastric plexus. Most of the sympathetic fibers are postganglionic efferent and afferent fibers. The external anal sphincter, a striated muscle, is innervated by the somatic pudendal nerves.

As in other regions of the gut, several diverse chemicals serve as mediators at presynaptic and postsynaptic junctions within the autonomic innervation to the large intestine. Acetylcholine (ACh) and tachykinins such as substance P serve as major excitatory mediators, and nitric oxide (NO), vasoactive intestinal peptide (VIP), and possibly adenosine triphosphate (ATP) serve as major inhibitory mediators. Transmission between the pudendal nerves and the external anal sphincter is mediated by ACh.

CONTRACTIONS OF THE CECUM AND ASCENDING COLON

The flow of contents from the small intestine into the large intestine is intermittent and is regulated partly by a sphincteric mechanism at the **ileocecal junction.** A sensor placed in the junction records pressures that are several millimeters of mercury (mm Hg) greater than those in the ileum or colon. The pressure is not constant, however; the sphincter relaxes periodically, and during this time ileal contractions propel contents into the large intestine (Fig. 6-2, *A*). Once material reaches the proximal large intestine, it is acted on by a wide variety of contractions. Most of these contractions are segmental, with durations of 12 to 60 seconds. The pressures generated by these contractions vary in amplitude, ranging between approximately 10 and 50 mm Hg.

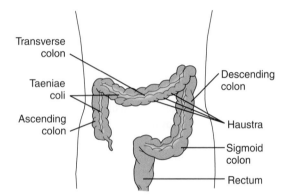

FIGURE 6-1 ■ Anatomy of the colon. The colon is shorter and of larger diameter than the small intestine. The longitudinal smooth muscle is concentrated into three bands (taeniae coli) in all regions except the rectum. Note that all regions except the rectum possess haustra. The exact cause of haustration is not known. Haustra are formed partly by contractions of the circular muscle; however, because they are still present after death, some investigators believe they have a permanent structural basis.

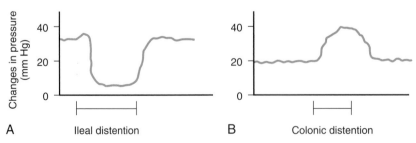

FIGURE 6-2 ■ Intraluminal pressures recorded at the level of the ileocecal sphincter. Note the resting pressure of 20 to 40 mm Hg. **A,** Distention of the ileum causes sphincteric relaxation and thus allows flow of contents from the ileum into the colon. **B,** Distention of the colon, by contrast, causes contraction of the sphincter to prevent passage of contents from the colon to the ileum. *(From Cohen S, Harris LD, Levitan R: Manometric characteristics of the human ileocecal junctional zone. Gastroenterology 54:72-75, 1968.)*

It is believed that these contractions are partly responsible for the haustrations seen in the colon. At adjacent sites, contractions usually occur independently. Thus they slowly move the contents back and forth, mixing and exposing them to the mucosa for absorption of water and electrolytes. In addition to pressure changes caused by segmental contractions, many of other pressure waves have been recorded. Attempts to classify these have been made, but the degree of overlap of pressure profiles makes classification difficult.

Occasionally, segmental contractions are organized in an oral-to-aboral direction; thus propulsion over short distances takes place. Usually, however, propulsion occurs during a characteristic sequence termed **mass movement.** Segmental activity suddenly ceases, and along with its disappearance is a loss of haustrations. The colon then undergoes a contraction

that sweeps intraluminal contents in an aboral direction (Fig. 6-3, *A* to *C*). After the mass movement, haustrations and phasic contractions return (Fig. 6-3, *D*). Mass movements are infrequent in healthy people and are estimated to occur only one to three times daily. Because they are such infrequent events, they have not been studied in any great detail in normal persons.

CONTRACTIONS OF THE DESCENDING AND SIGMOID COLON

By the time material reaches the descending and sigmoid colon, it has changed from a liquid to a semisolid state. Although there is less absorption of water and electrolytes from these portions of the colon, motility studies have demonstrated that contractions of the

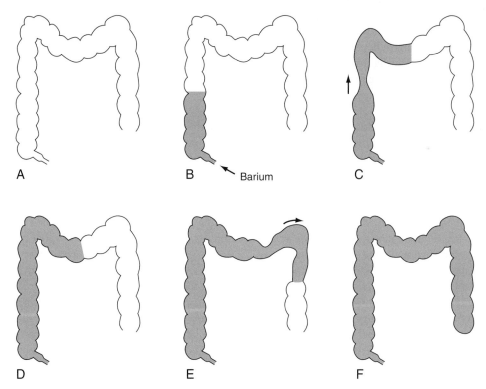

FIGURE 6-3 ■ Two mass movements. **A,** Appearance of the colon before the entry of barium sulfate. **B,** As the barium enters from the ileum, it is acted on by haustral contractions. **C,** As more barium enters, a portion is swept into and through an area of the colon that has lost its haustral markings. **D,** The barium is acted on by the returning haustral contractions. **E,** A second mass movement propels the barium into and through areas of the transverse and descending colon. **F,** Haustrations again return. This type of contraction accomplishes most of the movement of feces through the colon.

segmenting type are more frequent here than in the ascending and transverse colon. These segmenting contractions do not result in propulsion. On the contrary, they offer resistance and thus retard the flow of contents from more proximal regions into the rectum. Propulsion into and through these areas also occurs during mass movements. Here, too, there is a loss of segmental activity and the haustrations that precede transport (Fig. 6-3, *E* and *F*). Thus material that enters these regions during a mass movement is acted on to reduce its liquid content further and is then propelled into the rectum during a subsequent mass movement.

MOTILITY OF THE RECTUM AND ANAL CANAL

The rectum usually is empty or nearly so. Although very little material is present, contractions do occur in this region. In fact, the upper regions of the rectum contract segmentally more frequently than does the sigmoid colon. This activity tends to retard the flow of contents into the rectum. When the rectum fills, it does so intermittently. During a mass movement or during an aborally directed sequence of segmental contractions of the sigmoid colon, some material passes into the rectum.

Normally the anal canal is closed because of contraction of the internal anal sphincter. When the rectum is distended by fecal material, however, the internal sphincter relaxes as part of the **rectosphincteric reflex** (Fig. 6-4). Rectal distention also elicits a sensation that signals the urge for defecation. Defecation is prevented by the external anal sphincter, which is normally in a state of tonic contraction maintained by reflex activation through dorsal roots in the sacral segments. In paraplegic patients lacking this tonic contraction, the rectosphincteric reflex results in defecation. In the normal individual, if environmental conditions are not conducive to defecation, voluntary contractions of the external sphincter can overcome the reflex. Relaxation of the internal sphincter is transient because the receptors within the rectal wall accommodate the stimulus of distention. Thus the internal anal sphincter regains its tone, and the sensation subsides until the passage of more contents into the rectum. The rectum can accommodate rather large quantities of material, so it acts as a storage organ.

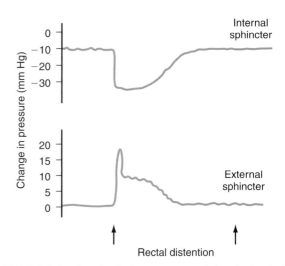

FIGURE 6-4 ■ Intraluminal pressure recorded at the level of the internal and external anal sphincters. Rectal distention causes relaxation of the internal sphincter and contraction of the external sphincter. Note, however, that the changes in sphincteric pressures are transient even though rectal distention is maintained. This finding is related to the accommodation of the stretch receptors within the wall of the rectum. *(Modified from Schuster MM, Hookman P, Hendrix TR: Simultaneous manometric recording of internal and external anal sphincteric reflexes. Johns Hopkins Med J 116: 70-88, 1965.)*

If the rectosphincteric reflex is elicited at a time when evacuation is convenient, defecation occurs. **Defecation** is accomplished by a series of voluntary and involuntary acts. When rectal distention is followed by defecation, muscles of the descending and sigmoid colon and the rectum may contract to propel contents toward the anal canal. Then both internal and external sphincters relax to allow passage of the bolus. Normally these events are accompanied by voluntary acts that raise intra-abdominal pressure and lower the pelvic floor. Intra-abdominal pressure is increased by contractions of the diaphragm and musculature of the abdominal wall. Simultaneously the musculature of the pelvic floor relaxes to allow the increased abdominal pressure to force the floor downward.

CONTROL OF MOTILITY

Factors that control motility of the large intestine are complex and poorly understood. As in the stomach and small intestine, motility in the large intestine is influenced by at least four factors: interstitial cells of Cajal–smooth muscle properties, enteric nerves, extrinsic nerves, and circulating or locally released chemicals.

The tone of the ileocecal sphincter is basically myogenic. It is modified, however, by nervous and humoral factors. Distention of the colon causes an increase in sphincteric tension, a reflex mediated by enteric nerves (see Fig. 6-2, *B*). Distention of the ileum causes relaxation, also mediated by enteric nerves (see Fig. 6-2, *A*). Relaxation of the sphincter and an increase in the contractile activity of the ileum occur with or shortly after eating. This has been termed the **gastroileal reflex.** One view is that the reflex is mediated by the gastrointestinal (GI) hormones, primarily gastrin and cholecystokinin (CCK). Both these hormones cause an increase in the contractile activity of the ileum, as well as relaxation of the ileocecal sphincter. Some investigators, however, think that this reflex is mediated via the extrinsic autonomic nerves to the intestine.

Smooth muscle cells of the ascending, transverse, descending, and sigmoid colon and of the rectum exhibit fluctuations in their membrane potential. Cyclic depolarizations and repolarizations that possess some of the characteristics of small intestinal slow waves can be recorded. As in the small intestine, these slow waves are thought to depend on interactions between smooth muscle cells and interstitial cells of Cajal. Potential changes that resemble spike potentials also are recorded. These changes probably initiate contractions, but the exact relationships between changes in potential and contractile activity have not been clarified. In addition, investigators have recorded various oscillations in membrane potential that fit descriptions of neither slow wave nor spike potential activities. The origin and function of these phenomena are less clear.

Enteric neurons are involved in the control of colonic contractions; aperistaltic reflex can be initiated in the colon, and this reflex is mediated by nerves within the myenteric plexus. These plexal nerves seem to be predominantly inhibitory because in their absence the colon is contracted tonically. Several colonic reflexes have their pathways in the extrinsic nerves. Distention of remote areas of the bowel induces an inhibition of contractions. The pathway for this reflex includes the inferior mesenteric ganglion and also may include the spinal cord. In addition, several investigations have demonstrated that emotional state has a marked influence on colonic motility. These influences of the central nervous system are mediated by the extrinsic nerves.

The GI hormones, as well as epinephrine and the prostaglandins, affect colonic motility. Gastrin and CCK increase colonic activity and have been implicated in the mass movement that sometimes occurs after eating. Epinephrine inhibits all contractile activity, whereas the prostaglandins (primarily E type) decrease segmenting contractions and increase propulsive activity. The importance of these agents in regulating colonic motility is not known.

The rectosphincteric reflex and the act of defecation are under neural control. Part of the control lies in the enteric nervous system. The reflex, however, is reinforced by activity of neurons within the spinal cord. Destruction of the nerves to the anorectal area can result in fecal retention. The sensation of rectal distention, as well as voluntary control of the external anal sphincter, is mediated by pathways within the spinal cord that lead to the cerebral cortex. Destruction of these pathways causes a loss of voluntary control of defecation.

CLINICAL SIGNIFICANCE

Abnormal transit of material through the colon is common. Delayed transit leads to **constipation;** in most situations, however, this is dietary in origin. There is a direct correlation among increased dietary fiber, increased colonic intraluminal bulk, and enhanced transit through the colon. How motility of the colon contributes to these changes in transit is not known. Laxatives work either by osmotic effects (polyethylene glycol, magnesium citrate, lactulose, and sorbitol) or by increasing

Continued

colonic propulsion (bisacodyl, sodium picosulfate, and glycerol). Alterations in motility and transit are frequently caused by emotional factors and are indicative of the strong influence of the higher centers of the central nervous system on motility. The final effects of stress on colonic motility vary greatly from individual to individual. Most students are familiar with diarrhea previous to an important examination. The severity of the problem is usually related inversely to how well the student is prepared for the test.

A particularly interesting and dramatic clinical disorder in which severe constipation is seen is congenital megacolon **(Hirschsprung's disease),** which is characterized by an absence of the enteric nervous system in the distal colon. The internal anal sphincter is always involved, and often the disease extends proximally into the rectum. The involved segment exhibits increased tone, has a very narrow lumen, and is devoid of propulsive activity. As a result, the colon proximal to the diseased segment becomes dilated, thus producing a megacolon. This condition is treated through surgical removal of the diseased segment.

In adults, the most common gastrointestinal disorder for which medical advice is sought is **irritable bowel syndrome.** This disorder gives rise most often to abdominal pain and altered bowel habit (constipation and/or diarrhea). In limited observations, exaggerated segmental contractions in the sigmoid colon have been seen, particularly in response to stimulants such as morphine. During stress, patients with irritable bowel syndrome and constipation exhibit increased segmentation in the sigmoid colon, whereas those with diarrhea exhibit decreased segmentation. In addition to motility disorders, sensory hypersensitivity to visceral stimulation may play a role. The cause of this disorder remains unknown. One theory suggests that altered motility may reflect the conditioning of autonomic responses from repeated exposure to stressful situations. Another suggests that gastrointestinal infections and alterations in normal colonic flora play a role in the origin of irritable bowel syndrome.

In older age groups, **diverticula** (outpouchings of mucosa that extend through the muscular wall) frequently develop in the colon. Evidence suggests that abnormal colonic motility leads to diverticulum formation because of the generation of increased intraluminal pressure. However, a direct correlation among abnormal motility, symptoms, and the presence of diverticula cannot always be demonstrated.

Despite the large numbers of patients in whom disordered colonic motility is suspected, techniques for monitoring contractions are not in general clinical use. Most often, radiologic procedures are used to provide limited information. In one test, radiopaque markers are ingested daily for 3 days. On the fourth day, a radiograph is taken, and the number of markers in each region of the colon is noted and compared with normal values. Measurements of intraluminal pressures and myoelectric activity are feasible, especially in the sigmoid colon and rectum, because these areas are readily accessible. To date, such techniques are mainly used in investigative studies.

The behavior of both the internal and the external anal sphincters, and the response to rectal distention, can be measured by the careful placement of two small intraluminal balloons in the anal canal. A third balloon is placed in the rectum and is distended to monitor the components of the defecation reflex. This technique is useful in patients with suspected neurologic disorders that result in impaired defecation.

SUMMARY

1. The muscular anatomy of the colon is characterized by concentration of the longitudinal muscle into bands called taeniae coli. Contraction of the taeniae coli and the circular muscle results in haustrations.

2. Most colonic contractions are of the segmenting type, which aid in the absorption of water and electrolytes. The frequency of segmenting contractions is higher in the descending and sigmoid colon than in areas located more orad. This retards aboral progression.

3. Aboral movement of contents is slow, usually taking days to pass material through the colon. Most aboral movement takes place during infrequent peristaltic contractions called mass movements.

4. Tonic contraction of the internal anal sphincter maintains closure of the anal canal. Distention of the rectum elicits relaxation of the internal anal sphincter and causes the urge to defecate. Defecation can be prevented by voluntary contraction of the external anal sphincter while the rectum accommodates to the distention and the internal anal sphincter regains its tone. Relaxation of the external anal sphincter during this time leads to defecation.

5. Colonic slow waves are cyclic depolarizations and repolarizations of muscle cell membranes that appear to set the timing of segmental contractions. Neural activity and hormone levels influence the intensity of segmental contractions.

6. Mass movements are regulated by activities of the intrinsic and extrinsic nerves and possibly by the hormones gastrin and CCK. The rectosphincteric reflex is regulated by intrinsic, extrinsic autonomic, and somatic nerves.

KEY WORDS AND CONCEPTS

Cecum	Shunt fascicles
Ascending/transverse/descending/sigmoid colon	Ileocecal junction
	Mass movement
Rectum	Rectosphincteric reflex
Anal canal	Defecation
Taeniae coli	Gastroileal reflex
Internal anal sphincter	Constipation
External anal sphincter	Hirschsprung's disease
Haustra/haustrations	Irritable bowel syndrome
	Diverticula

SUGGESTED READINGS

Bharucha AE, Brookes SJH: Neurophysiologic mechanisms of human large intestinal motility. In Johnson LR, editor: ed 5, *Physiology of the Gastrointestinal Tract*, vol 1, San Diego, 2012, Elsevier.

Christensen J: The motility of the colon. In Johnson LR, editor: ed 3, *Physiology of the Gastrointestinal Tract*, vol 1, New York, 1994, Raven Press.

Phillips SF: Motility disorders of the colon. In Yamada T, Alpers DH, Laine L, et al: ed 3, *Textbook of Gastroenterology*, vol 1, Philadelphia, 1999, Lippincott Williams & Wilkins.

Sarna S: Large intestinal motility. In Johnson LR, editor: ed 4, *Physiology of the Gastrointestinal Tract*, vol 1, San Diego, 2006, Elsevier.

SALIVARY SECRETION

OBJECTIVES

- Discuss the constituents and various functions of saliva.
- Understand the mechanisms leading to the formation of saliva.
- Explain the processes resulting in the tonicity of saliva and concentrations of its various ions.
- Describe the regulation of salivary secretion.

Although the salivary glands are not essential to life, their secretions are important for the hygiene and comfort of the mouth and teeth. The functions of saliva may be divided into those concerned with **lubrication, protection,** and **digestion.** An active process produces saliva in large quantities relative to the weight of the salivary glands. Saliva is hyposmotic at all rates of secretion, and in contrast to the other gastrointestinal (GI) secretions, the rate of secretion is almost totally under the control of the nervous system. Another characteristic of this regulation is that both branches of the autonomic nervous system (ANS) stimulate secretion. However, the parasympathetic system provides a much greater stimulus than does the sympathetic system.

FUNCTIONS OF SALIVA

The lubricating ability of saliva depends primarily on its content of **mucus.** In the mouth, mixing saliva with food lubricates the ingested material and facilitates the swallowing process. The lubricating effect of saliva is also necessary for speech, as evidenced by the glass of water normally found on the podium of a public speaker.

Saliva exerts its effects through a variety of different mechanisms. It protects the mouth by buffering and diluting noxious substances. Hot solutions of tea, coffee, or soup, for example, are diluted and cooled by saliva. Foul-tasting substances can be washed from the mouth by copious salivation. Similarly, the salivary glands are stimulated strongly before vomiting. The corrosive gastric acid and pepsin that are brought up into the esophagus and mouth are thereby neutralized and diluted by saliva. Dry mouth, or xerostomia, is associated with chronic infections of the buccal mucosa and with dental caries. Saliva dissolves and washes out food particles from between the teeth. Certain specialized constituents of saliva have antibacterial actions. These include the following: a **lysozyme,** which attacks bacterial cell walls; **lactoferrin,** which chelates iron and thus prevents the multiplication of organisms that require it for growth; and the **binding glycoprotein for immunoglobulin A** (IgA), which in combination with IgA forms secretory IgA, which in turn is immunologically active against viruses and bacteria. Various inorganic compounds are taken up by the salivary glands, concentrated, and secreted in saliva. These include fluoride and calcium (Ca^{2+}), which are subsequently incorporated into the teeth.

The contributions made by saliva to normal digestion include dissolving and washing away food particles on the taste buds to enable one to taste the next morsel of food eaten. Saliva contains two enzymes, one directed toward carbohydrates and the other toward fat. An **α-amylase** called **ptyalin** cleaves internal α-1,4-glycosidic bonds present in starch. Exhaustive digestion of starch by this enzyme, identical to pancreatic amylase, produces maltose, maltotriose, and α-limit dextrins, which contain the α-1,6 branch points of the original molecule. Salivary amylase has a pH optimum of 7, and it is rapidly denatured at pH 4. However, because a large portion of a meal often remains unmixed for a considerable length of time in the orad stomach, the salivary enzyme may account for the digestion of as much as 75% of the starch present before it is denatured by gastric acid. In the absence of salivary amylase, there is no defect in carbohydrate digestion because the pancreatic enzyme is secreted in amounts sufficient to digest all the starch present.

The serous salivary glands of the tongue secrete the second digestive enzyme, **lingual lipase,** which plays a role in the hydrolysis of dietary lipid. Unlike pancreatic lipase, lingual lipase has properties that allow it to act in all parts of the upper GI tract. Thus the ability of lingual lipase to hydrolyze lipids is not affected by surface-active detergents such as bile salts, medium chain fatty acids, and lecithin. It has an acidic pH optimum and remains active through the stomach and into the intestine.

ANATOMY AND INNERVATION OF THE SALIVARY GLANDS

The salivary glands are a collection of somewhat dissimilar structures in the mouth that produce a common juice (the saliva), although the composition of the secretion from different salivary glands varies. The largest of the salivary structures are the paired **parotid glands,** located near the angle of the jaw and the ear. They are serous glands, secrete a fairly watery juice rich in amylase, and account for approximately 25% of the daily output of saliva. The smaller bilateral **submandibular** and **sublingual glands** are mixed glands, containing both serous and mucous cells. They elaborate a more viscid saliva and secrete most of the remaining 75% of the output. Other, still smaller glands are present in the mucosa covering the palate, buccal areas, lips, and tongue.

Most of the salivary glands are ectodermal in origin. The combined secretion of the parotid and submandibular glands constitutes 90% of the volume of saliva, which in a normal adult can amount to a liter daily. The specific gravity of this mixed juice ranges from 1.000 to 1.010.

The microscopic structure of the salivary glands combines many features observed in another exocrine gland, the pancreas. A salivary gland consists of a blind-end system of microscopic ducts that branch out from grossly visible ducts. One main duct opens into the mouth from each gland. The functional unit of the salivary duct system, the **salivon,** is depicted in Figure 7-1. At the blind end is the **acinus,** surrounded by polygonal acinar cells. These cells secrete the initial saliva, including water, electrolytes, and organic molecules such as amylase. The solutes and fluid move out of the acinar cell into the duct lumen to form the initial saliva. The acinar cells are surrounded in turn by **myoepithelial cells.** The myoepithelial cells rest on the basement membrane of acinar cells. They contain an actinomycin and have motile extensions. The next segment of the salivon is the **intercalated duct,** which may be associated with additional myoepithelial cells. Contraction of myoepithelial cells serves to expel formed saliva from the acinus, oppose retrograde movement of the juice during active secretion of saliva, shorten and widen the internal diameter of the intercalated duct (thereby lowering resistance to the flowing saliva), and prevent distention of the acinus (distention of the blind end of the salivon would permit back-diffusion of formed saliva through the stretched surface of the acinus). Thus the myoepithelial cells support the acinus against the increased intraluminal pressures that occur during secretion.

Whenever there is an abrupt need for saliva in the mouth (e.g., immediately before vomiting), myoepithelial cell contraction propels the secretion into the main duct of the gland. Other exocrine glands, such as the mammary glands and the pancreas, also possess myoepithelial cells.

The intercalated duct soon widens to become the **striated duct,** lined by columnar epithelial cells that resemble the epithelial components of the renal tubule in both shape and function. The saliva in the intercalated duct is similar in ionic composition to plasma. Changes from that composition occur because of ion exchanges in the striated duct. As saliva traverses the striated duct, sodium (Na^+) is actively reabsorbed from the juice, and potassium (K^+) is transported into it. Ca^{2+} also enters secreting duct cells during salivation. Similarly, anionic exchange occurs; chloride

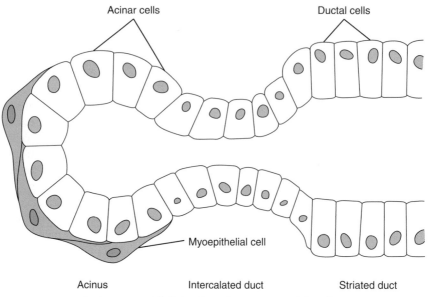

Acinar cells

Ductal cells

Myoepithelial cell

Acinus   Intercalated duct   Striated duct

FIGURE 7-1 ■ Cells lining the various portions of the salivon.

(Cl⁻) is reabsorbed from the saliva, and bicarbonate (HCO_3^-) is added to it.

The striated duct epithelium is considered to be a fairly "tight" sheet membrane. That is, its surface is fairly impermeable to the back-diffusion of water from the saliva into the tissue, and osmotic gradients develop between the saliva and interstitial fluid through the reabsorption of Na^+ and Cl^-. The result is hypotonic saliva.

The blood supplied to the salivary glands is distributed by branches of the external carotid artery. The direction of arterial flow within each salivary gland is opposite the direction of flowing saliva within the ducts of each salivon. The arterioles break up into capillaries around the acini, as well as in nonacinar areas. Blood from nonacinar areas passes through portal venules back to the acinar capillaries, from which a second set of venules then drains all the blood to the systemic venous circulation. The rate of blood flow through resting salivary tissue is approximately 20 times that through muscle. This blood flow in part accounts for the prodigious amounts of saliva produced relative to the weight of the glands.

Both components of the ANS reach the salivary glands. The parasympathetic preganglionic fibers are delivered by the facial and glossopharyngeal nerves to autonomic ganglia, from which the postganglionic fibers pass to individual glands. The sympathetic preganglionic nerves originate at the cervical ganglion, whose postganglionic fibers extend to the glands in the periarterial spaces (these relationships appear in Fig. 7-2). Parasympathetic and sympathetic mediators regulate all known salivary gland functions to an extraordinary degree. Their influence includes major effects, not only on secretion but also on blood flow, ductular smooth muscle activity, growth, and metabolism of the salivary glands.

COMPOSITION OF SALIVA

The major constituents of saliva are water, electrolytes, and a few enzymes. The **unique properties** of this GI juice are (1) its large volume relative to the mass of glands that secrete saliva, (2) its low osmolality, (3) its high K^+ concentration, and (4) the specific organic materials it contains.

Inorganic Composition

Compared with other secretory organs of the GI tract, the salivary glands elaborate a remarkably large volume of juice per gram (g) of tissue. Thus, for example, an entire pancreas may reach a maximal rate of

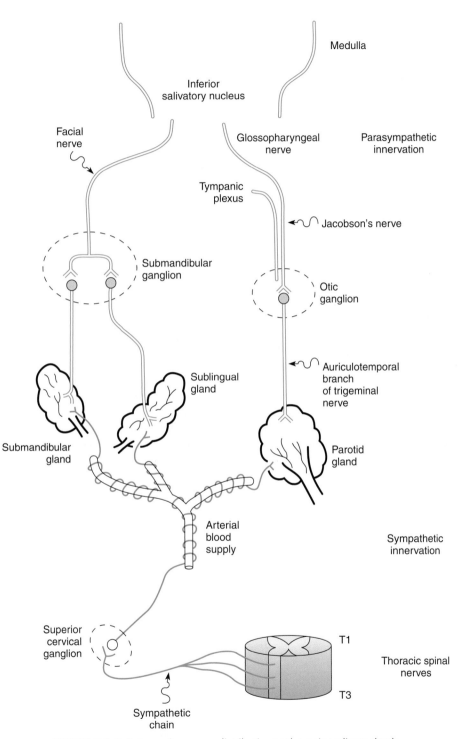

FIGURE 7-2 ■ Autonomic nervous distribution to the major salivary glands.

secretion of 1 milliliter (mL)/minute, whereas at the highest rates of secretion in some animals, a tiny submaxillary gland can secrete 1 mL/g/minute, a 50-fold higher rate. In humans, the salivary glands secrete at rates severalfold higher than other GI organs per unit weight of tissue.

The osmolality of saliva is significantly lower than that of plasma at all but the highest rates of secretion, when the saliva becomes isotonic with plasma. As the secretory rate of the salivon increases, the osmolality of its saliva also increases.

The concentrations of electrolytes in saliva vary with the rate of secretion (Fig. 7-3). The K^+ concentration of saliva is 2 to 30 times that of the plasma, depending on the rate of secretion, the nature of the stimulus, the plasma K^+ concentration, and the level of mineralocorticoids in the circulation. Saliva has the highest K^+ concentration of any digestive juice; maximal concentration values approach those within cells. These remarkable levels of salivary K^+ imply the existence of an energy-dependent transport mechanism within the salivon. In most species the concentration of Na^+ in saliva is always less than that in plasma, and, as the secretory rate increases, the Na^+ concentration also increases. In general, Cl^- concentrations parallel those of Na^+. These findings suggest that Na^+ and Cl^- are secreted and then reabsorbed as the saliva passes through the ducts. The concentration of HCO_3^- in saliva is higher than that in plasma, except at low flow rates. This also accounts for the changes in the pH of saliva. At basal rates of flow the pH is slightly acidic but rapidly rises to approximately 8 as flow is stimulated. The relationships between ion concentrations and flow rates (shown in Fig. 7-3) vary somewhat, depending on the stimulus.

The relationships shown in Figure 7-3 are explained by two basic types of studies that indicate how the final saliva is produced. First, fluid collected by micropuncture of the intercalated ducts contains Na^+, K^+, Cl^-, and HCO_3^- in concentrations approximately equal to their plasma concentrations. This fluid also is isotonic to plasma. Second, if one perfuses a salivary gland duct with fluid containing ions in concentrations similar to those of plasma, Na^+ and Cl^- concentrations are decreased and K^+ and HCO_3^- concentrations are increased when the fluid is collected at the duct opening. The fluid also becomes hypotonic, and the longer the fluid remains in the duct (i.e., the slower the rate of perfusion), the greater are the changes. These data indicate, first, that the acini secrete a fluid similar to plasma in its concentration of ions and, second, that as the fluid moves down the duct, Na^+ and Cl^- are reabsorbed and K^+ and HCO_3^- are secreted into the saliva. The higher the flow of saliva, the less time is available

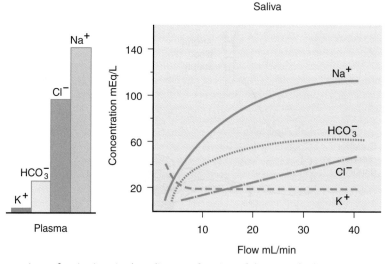

FIGURE 7-3 ▪ Concentrations of major ions in the saliva as a function of the rate of salivary secretion. Values in plasma are shown for comparison. Cl^-, chloride; HCO_3^-, bicarbonate; K^+, potassium; Na^+, sodium.

for modification, and the final saliva more closely resembles plasma in its ionic makeup (see Fig. 7-3). At low flow rates K^+ increases considerably, and Na^+ and Cl^- decrease. Because most salivary agonists stimulate HCO_3^- secretion, the HCO_3^- concentration remains relatively high, even at high rates of secretion. Some K^+ and HCO_3^- are reabsorbed in exchange for Na^+ and Cl^-, but much more Na^+ and Cl^- leave the duct, thus causing the saliva to become hypotonic. Because the duct epithelium is relatively impermeable to water, the final product remains hypotonic. These processes are depicted in Figure 7-4.

Current evidence indicates that Cl^- is the primary ion that is actively secreted by the acinar cells (Fig. 7-5). No evidence exists for direct active secretion of Na^+. The secretory mechanism for Cl^- is inhibited by ouabain, a finding indicating that it depends on the Na^+/K^+ pump in the basolateral membrane. The active pumping of Na^+ out of the cell creates a diffusion gradient for Na^+ to enter across the basolateral membrane. Two main ion transport pathways exploit this Na^+ gradient to accumulate Cl^- above its equilibrium potential. In the first (see Fig. 7-5, cell 1), $2Cl^-$ are cotransported with Na^+ and K^+ into the cell to preserve electrical neutrality. This process increases the electrochemical potential of Cl^- within the cell, and Cl^- diffuses down this gradient into the lumen via an electrogenic ion channel that may also allow HCO_3^- to enter the lumen. Inhibition of the $Na^+/K^+/2Cl^-$ cotransporter decreases salivary secretion by 65%. In the second (see Fig. 7-5, cell 2), Na^+ enters in exchange for hydrogen (H^+), which alkalinizes the cell promoting the intracellular accumulation of HCO_3^-, which

then is exchanged for Cl^-. Removal of HCO_3^- from the perfusate or inhibition of the Na^+/H^+ exchanger by amiloride reduces secretion by 30%. In both cases Na^+ moves paracellularly through the tight junctions and into the lumen, thus preserving electroneutrality; water follows down its osmotic gradient. Evidence indicates that water also moves into the saliva transcellularly through the aquaporin 5 apical water channel. There may also be a Ca^{2+}-activated K^+ channel in the basolateral membrane. Exodus of K^+ increases the electronegativity of the cytosol and thereby increases the driving force for the entry of Cl^- and HCO_3^- into the lumen. Agents that stimulate salivary secretion increase the activity of all these channels and transport processes.

Within the ducts, Na^+ and Cl^- are actively absorbed and K^+ and HCO_3^- are actively secreted (Fig. 7-6). These processes are also inhibited by ouabain and depend on the Na^+ gradient created by the Na^+, K^+-adenosine triphosphatase (ATPase) in the basolateral membrane. The apical membrane contains a Na^+ channel, and its movement into the cell supports the electrogenic movement of Cl^- into the cell through Cl^- channels. The Na/K-ATPase pumps Na^+ out while a Cl^- channel in the basolateral membrane transports it out of the cell. Cl^- reabsorption also occurs via the paracellular pathway. K^+ is secreted through apical channels into the saliva. To secrete HCO_3^- into the lumen, HCO_3^- must be concentrated within the cell. This occurs via an Na/HCO_3^- transporter in the basolateral membrane, which is driven by the Na^+ gradient. HCO_3^- leaves the cell either through the apical cyclic adenosine monophosphate (cAMP)-activated **CFTR (cystic fibrosis transmembrane regulator)** Cl^- channel or via the Cl^-/HCO_3^-

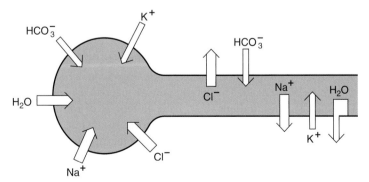

FIGURE 7-4 ■ Movements of ions and water (H_2O) in the acinus and duct of the salivon. Cl^-, chloride; HCO_3^-, bicarbonate; K^+, potassium; Na^+, sodium.

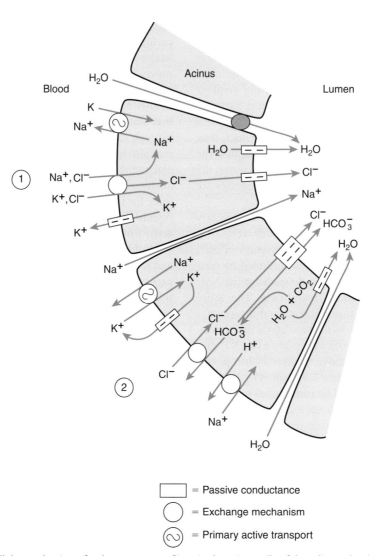

FIGURE 7-5 ■ Intracellular mechanisms for the movement of ions in the acinar cells of the salivary glands. Cl^-, chloride; HCO_3^-, bicarbonate; H_2O, water; K^+, potassium; Na^+, sodium.

exchanger at the apical membrane. The tight junctions of the ductule epithelium are relatively impermeable to water when compared with those of the acini. The net results are a decrease in Na^+ and Cl^- concentrations and an increase in K^+ and HCO_3^- concentrations, as well as pH, as the saliva moves down the duct. More ions leave than water (H_2O), and the saliva becomes hypotonic. Aldosterone acts at the luminal membrane to increase the absorption of Na^+ and the secretion of K^+ by increasing the numbers of their channels.

Organic Composition

Some organic materials produced and secreted by the salivary glands are mentioned earlier in the section on the functions of saliva. These materials include the enzymes α-amylase (ptyalin) and lingual lipase, mucus, glycoproteins, lysozymes, and lactoferrin. Another enzyme produced by salivary glands is **kallikrein,** which converts a plasma protein into the potent vasodilator **bradykinin.** Kallikrein is released when the metabolism of the salivary glands increases; it is

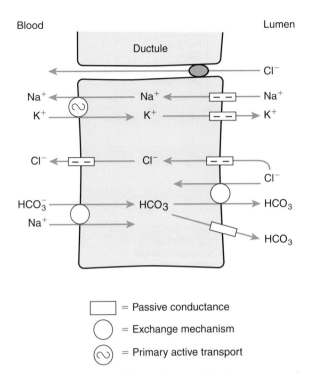

Blood   Lumen

FIGURE 7-6 ■ Intracellular mechanisms for the movement of ions in ductule cells of the salivary glands. Cl^-, chloride; HCO_3^-, bicarbonate; K^+, potassium; Na^+, sodium.

responsible in part for increased blood flow to the secreting glands. Saliva also contains the blood group substances A, B, AB, and O.

The synthesis of salivary gland enzymes, their storage, and their release are similar to the same processes in the pancreas (detailed in Chapter 9). The protein concentration of saliva is approximately one tenth the concentration of proteins in the plasma.

REGULATION OF SALIVARY SECRETION

The ANS controls essentially all salivary gland secretion. Antidiuretic hormone (ADH), or vasopressin, and aldosterone modify the composition of saliva by decreasing its Na^+ concentration and increasing its K^+ concentration, but they do not regulate the flow of saliva. The absence of hormonal control of salivation contrasts with the regulation of the flow of gastric and pancreatic juice and bile. The GI hormones exert major influences on the secretory activity of the

stomach, pancreas, and liver. Control of the salivary glands is also unusual in that both the parasympathetic and sympathetic branches stimulate secretion. The parasympathetic system, however, exerts a much greater influence.

Stimulation of the parasympathetic nerves to the salivary glands begins and maintains salivary secretion. Increased secretion results from the activation of transport processes in both acinar and duct cells. Secretion is enhanced by the contraction of the myoepithelial cells that are innervated by the parasympathetic nerves. Parasympathetic fibers also innervate the surrounding blood vessels, thus stimulating vasodilation and increasing blood flow to the secreting cells. Increased cellular activity in response to parasympathetic stimulation results in higher consumption of glucose and oxygen and in the production of vasodilator metabolites. In addition, kallikrein is released, resulting in the production of the vasodilator bradykinin. Increased cellular activity eventually leads to growth of the salivary glands. Section of the parasympathetic nerves to the salivary glands causes the glands to atrophy. These processes are outlined in Figure 7-7.

Sympathetic activation also stimulates secretion, myoepithelial cell contraction, metabolism, and growth of the salivary glands, although these effects are less pronounced and of shorter duration than are those produced by the parasympathetic nerves. Stimulation via the sympathetic nerves produces a biphasic change in blood flow to the salivary glands. The earliest response is a decrease caused by activation of α-adrenergic receptors and vasoconstriction. However, as vasodilator metabolites are produced, blood flow increases over resting levels. Section of the sympathetic fibers to the salivary glands, unlike section of the parasympathetic fibers, has little effect. The effects of sympathetic stimulation also are summarized in Figure 7-7.

Salivary glands contain receptors to many mediators, but the most important functionally are the muscarinic cholinergic and β-adrenergic receptors. The parasympathetic mediator is acetylcholine (ACh), which acts on muscarinic receptors and thereby results in the formation of inositol triphosphate (IP$_3$) and the subsequent release of Ca^{2+} from intracellular stores. Ca^{2+} also may enter the cell from outside. Other agents that are released from neurons in salivary glands and

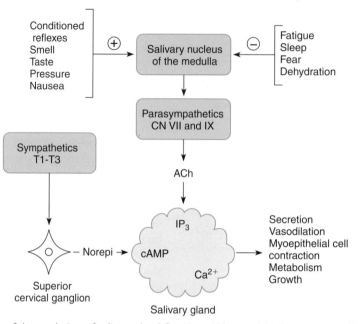

FIGURE 7-7 ■ Summary of the regulation of salivary gland function. ACh, acetylcholine; cAMP, cyclic adenosine monophosphate; Ca²⁺, calcium; CN, cranial nerve; IP₃, inositol triphosphate; Norepi, norepinephrine.

that release Ca^{2+} include vasoactive intestinal peptide (VIP) and substance P. The primary sympathetic mediator is norepinephrine, which binds to β-adrenergic receptors, a process resulting in the formation of cAMP. Formation of these second messengers causes protein phosphorylation and enzyme activation that ultimately leads to the stimulation of the salivary glands. In general, agonists that release Ca^{2+} have a greater effect on the volume of acinar cell secretion, whereas those elevating cAMP lead to a greater increase in enzyme and mucus content.

The dual autonomic regulation of the salivary glands is unusual in that both the parasympathetic and sympathetic systems stimulate secretory, metabolic, trophic, muscular, and circulatory functions in similar directions. Their complementary effects are shown in Figure 7-7.

Ultimately, the central nervous system and its autonomic arms are what respond to external events and either stimulate or inhibit activities of the salivary glands. Common events leading to increased glandular activities include chewing, consuming spicy or sour-tasting foods, and smoking. External events leading to glandular inhibition include sleep, fear, dehydration, and fatigue. Glandular activities sensitive to neural control include secretion, circulation, myoepithelial contraction, cellular metabolism, and even parenchymal growth.

CLINICAL CORRELATION

Medical conditions can alter either the amount or the composition of saliva. Mumps is a common childhood infection of the salivary glands that results in swelling, which can affect salivation. Besides congenital xerostomia (absence of saliva), there is Sjögren's syndrome, an acquired disease characterized by atrophy of the glands and decreased salivation. The commonly used drugs of the digitalis family cause increased concentrations of calcium and potassium in saliva. In patients with

SUMMARY

1. The functions of saliva include those concerned with digestion, protection, and lubrication.

2. Saliva is noteworthy in that it is produced in large volumes relative to the weight of the glands, is hypotonic, and contains relatively high concentrations of K^+.

3. The primary saliva is produced in end pieces called acini and is then modified as it passes through the ducts.

4. Acinar secretion contains ions and water in concentrations approximately equal to those in plasma.

5. Within the ducts, Na^+ and Cl^- are reabsorbed, and K^+ and HCO_3^- are secreted.

6. Because the ductule epithelium is relatively impermeable to water and ions, the saliva becomes more hypotonic as it moves through the ducts.

7. All regulatory control of salivation is provided by the ANS, and both the parasympathetic and sympathetic branches stimulate secretion and metabolism of the glands.

KEY WORDS AND CONCEPTS

Lubrication

Protection

Digestion

Mucus

Lysozyme

Lactoferrin

Binding glycoprotein for immunoglobulin A

α-Amylase

Ptyalin

Lingual lipase

Parotid glands

Submandibular/sublingual glands

Salivon

Acinus

Myoepithelial cells

Intercalated duct

Striated duct

Unique properties

Kallikrein

Bradykinin

SUGGESTED READINGS

Cook DI, van Lennep EW, Roberts M, et al: Secretion by the major salivary glands. In Johnson LR, editor: ed 3, *Physiology of the Gastrointestinal Tract*, vol 2, New York, 1994, Raven Press.

Melvin JE, Culp DJ: Salivary glands, physiology. In Johnson LR, editor: *Encyclopedia of Gastroenterology*, vol 3, San Diego, 2004, Academic Press, pp 318–325.

Catalan MA, Ambatipudi KS, Melvin JE: Salivary gland secretion. In Johnson LR, editor: ed 5, *Physiology of the Gastrointestinal Tract*, vol 2, San Diego, 2012, Elsevier.

8 GASTRIC SECRETION

OBJECTIVES

- Identify the secretory products of the stomach, their cells of origin, and their functions.
- Understand the mechanisms making it possible for the stomach to secrete 150 mN hydrochloric acid.
- Describe the electrolyte composition of gastric secretion and how it varies with the rate of secretion.
- Identify the major stimulants of the parietal cell and explain their interactions.
- Discuss the phases involved in the stimulation of gastric acid secretion and the processes acting in each.
- Identify factors that both stimulate and inhibit the release of the hormone gastrin.
- Explain the processes that result in the inhibition of gastric acid secretion following the ingestion of a meal and its emptying from the stomach.
- Describe the processes resulting in gastric and duodenal ulcer diseases.

Five constituents of gastric juice—**intrinsic factor, hydrogen ion** (H^+), **pepsin, mucus, and water**—have physiologic functions. They are secreted by the various cells present within the gastric mucosa. The only indispensable ingredient in gastric juice is intrinsic factor, required for the absorption of vitamin B_{12} by the ileal mucosa. Acid is necessary for the conversion of inactive pepsinogen to the enzyme pepsin. Acid and pepsin begin the digestion of protein, but in their absence pancreatic enzymes hydrolyze all ingested protein, so no nitrogen is wasted in the stools. Acid also kills a large number of bacteria that enter the stomach, thereby reducing the number of organisms reaching the intestine. In cases of severely reduced or absent acid secretion, the incidence of intestinal infections is greater. Mucus lines the wall of the stomach and protects it from damage. Mucus acts primarily as a lubricant, protecting the mucosa from physical injury. Together with bicarbonate (HCO_3^-), mucus neutralizes acid and maintains the surface of the mucosa at a pH near neutrality. This is part of the **gastric mucosal barrier** that protects the stomach from acid and pepsin digestion. Water acts as the medium for the action of acid and enzymes and solubilizes many of the constituents of a meal.

Gastric juice and many of its functions originally were described by a young army surgeon, William Beaumont, stationed at a fort on Mackinac Island in northern Michigan. Beaumont was called to treat a French Canadian, Alexis St. Martin, who had been accidentally shot in the side at close range with a shotgun. St. Martin unexpectedly survived but was left with a permanent opening into his stomach from the outside (gastric fistula). The accident occurred in 1822, and during the ensuing 3 years Beaumont nursed St. Martin back to health. Beaumont retained St. Martin "for the purpose of making physiological experiments," which were begun in 1825. Beaumont's observations and conclusions, many of which remain unchanged today, include the description of the juice itself and its digestive and bacteriostatic functions, the identification of the acid as hydrochloric, the realization that mucus was a separate secretion, the realization that mental disturbances affected gastric function, a direct study of gastric motility, and a thorough study of the ability of gastric juices to digest various foodstuffs.

FUNCTIONAL ANATOMY

Functionally, the gastric mucosa is divided into the **oxyntic gland area** and the **pyloric gland area** (Fig. 8-1). The oxyntic gland mucosa secretes acid and is located in the proximal 80% of the stomach. It includes the body and the fundus. The distal 20% of the gastric mucosa, referred to as the *pyloric gland mucosa,* synthesizes and releases the hormone gastrin. This area of the stomach often is designated the **antrum.**

The gastric mucosa is composed of pits and glands (Fig. 8-2). The pits and surface itself are lined with mucous or surface epithelial cells. At the base of the pits are the openings of the glands, which project into the mucosa toward the outside or serosa. The oxyntic glands contain the acid-producing **parietal cells** and the **peptic** or **chief cells,** which secrete the enzyme precursor **pepsinogen.** Pyloric glands contain the gastrin-producing G cells and mucous cells, which also produce pepsinogen. Mucous neck cells are present where the glands open into the pits. Each gland contains a stem cell in this region. These cells divide; one daughter cell remains anchored as the stem cell, and the other divides several times. The resulting new cells migrate both to the surface, where they differentiate into mucous cells, and down into the glands, where they become parietal cells in the oxyntic gland area. Endocrine cells such as the G cells also differentiate from stem cells. Peptic cells are capable of mitosis, but evidence indicates that they also can arise from stem cells during the repair of damage to the mucosa. Cells of the surface and pits are replaced much more rapidly than are those of the glands.

The parietal cells secrete hydrochloric acid (HCl) and, in humans, intrinsic factor. In some species the chief cells also secrete intrinsic factor. The normal human stomach contains approximately 1 billion parietal cells, which produce acid at a concentration of 150 to 160 mEq/L. The number of parietal cells determines the maximal secretory rate and accounts for interindividual variability. The human stomach secretes 1 to 2 L of gastric juice per day. Because the pH of the final juice at high rates of secretion may be less than 1 and that of the blood is 7.4, the parietal cells must expend a large amount of energy to concentrate H^+. The energy for the production of this more than a million fold concentration gradient comes from adenosine triphosphate (ATP), which is produced by the numerous mitochondria located within the cell (Fig. 8-3).

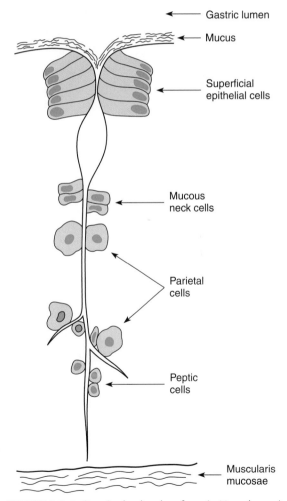

FIGURE 8-2 ■ Oxyntic gland and surface pit. Note the positions of the various cell types.

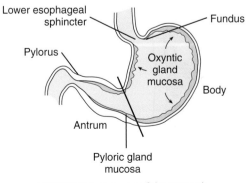

FIGURE 8-1 ■ Areas of the stomach.

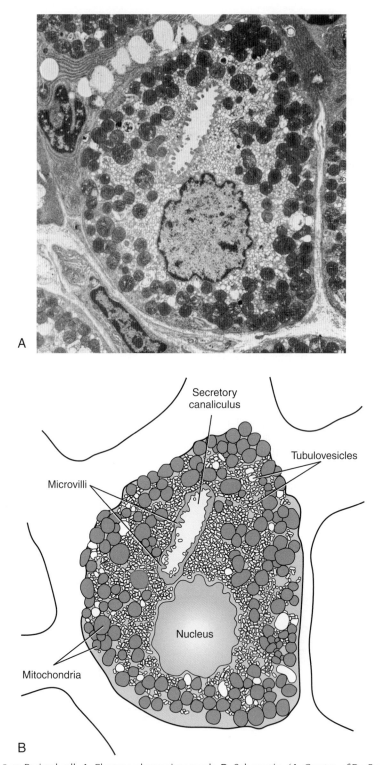

FIGURE 8-3 ■ Parietal cell. **A,** Electron photomicrograph. **B,** Schematic. *(**A,** Courtesy of Dr. Bruce MacKay.)*

During the resting state, the cytoplasm of the parietal cells is dominated by numerous **tubulovesicles.** There is also an **intracellular canaliculus** that is continuous with the lumen of the oxyntic gland. The tubulovesicles contain the enzymes **carbonic anhydrase** (CA) and **H+, potassium (K+)-ATPase** (H+,K+-ATPase), necessary for the production and secretion of acid, on their apical membranes. Thus, in the resting parietal cell, any basal secretion is directed into the lumen of the tubulovesicles and not into the cytoplasm of the cell. Stimulation of acid secretion causes the migration of the tubulovesicles and their incorporation into the membrane of the canaliculus as microvilli. As a result, the surface area of the canaliculus is greatly expanded to occupy much of the cell. The activities of the enzymes, which are now in the canalicular membrane, increase significantly during acid secretion. Acid secretion begins within 10 minutes of administering a stimulant. This lag time probably is expended in the morphologic conversion and enzyme activations described previously. Following the removal of stimulation, the tubulovesicles reform and the canaliculus regains its resting configuration.

The surface epithelial mucous cells are recognized primarily by the large number of mucous granules at their apical surfaces. During secretion, the membranes of the granules fuse with the cell membrane and expel mucus.

Peptic cells contain a highly developed endoplasmic reticulum for the synthesis of pepsinogen. The proenzyme is packaged into zymogen granules by the numerous Golgi structures within the cytoplasm. The zymogen granules migrate to the apical surface, where, during secretion, they empty their contents into the lumen by exocytosis. This entire procedure of enzyme synthesis, packaging, and secretion is discussed in greater detail in Chapter 9.

Endocrine cells of the gut also contain numerous granules. Unlike in the peptic and mucous cells, however, these hormone-containing granules are located at the base of the cell. The hormones are secreted into the intercellular space, from which they diffuse into the capillaries. The endocrine cells have numerous microvilli extending from their apical surface into the lumen. Presumably the microvilli contain receptors that sample the luminal contents and trigger hormone secretion in response to the appropriate stimuli.

SECRETION OF ACID

The transport processes involved in the secretion of HCl are shown in Figure 8-4. The exact biochemical steps for the production of H+ are not known, but the reaction can be summarized as follows:

$$HOH \rightarrow OH^- + H^+ \tag{1}$$

$$OH^- + CO_2 \xrightarrow{CA} HCO_3^- \tag{2}$$

H+ is pumped actively into the lumen and HCO_3^- diffuses into the blood, thus giving gastric venous blood a higher pH than that of arterial blood when the stomach is secreting. Step 2 is catalyzed by CA. Inhibition of this enzyme decreases the rate but does not prevent acid secretion. Metabolism produces much of the carbon dioxide (CO_2) used to neutralize hydroxyl (OH^-), but at high secretory rates, CO_2 from the blood also is required. The active transport of H+ across the mucosal membrane is catalyzed by H+,K+-ATPase, and H+ is pumped into the lumen in exchange for K+. Within the cell, K+ is accumulated by the sodium (Na+),K+-ATPase in the basolateral membrane. Accumulated K+ moves down its electrochemical gradient and leaks across both membranes. Luminal K+ is therefore recycled by the H+,K+-ATPase.

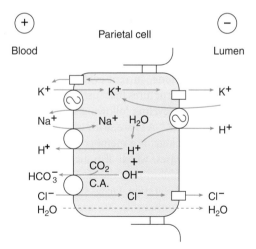

FIGURE 8-4 ▪ Transport processes in the gastric mucosa accounting for the presence of the various ions in gastric juice and for the negative transmembrane potential. C.A., carbonic anhydrase; Cl−, chloride; CO_2, carbon dioxide; H+, hydrogen ion; HCO_3^-, bicarbonate; H_2O, water; K+, potassium; Na+, sodium; OH−, hydroxyl.

Chloride (Cl^-) enters the cell across the basolateral membrane in exchange for HCO_3^-. The pumping of H^+ out of the cell allows OH^- to accumulate and form HCO_3^- from CO_2, a step catalyzed by CA. The HCO_3^- entering the blood causes the blood's pH to increase, so the gastric venous blood from the actively secreting stomach has a higher pH than arterial blood. The production of OH^- is facilitated by the low intracellular Na^+ concentration established by the Na^+,K^+-ATPase. Some Na^+ moves down its gradient back into the cell in exchange for H^+, thus further increasing OH^- production. This process in turn increases HCO_3^- production and enhances the driving force for the entry of Cl^- and its uphill movement from the blood into the lumen. Thus the movement of Cl^- from blood to lumen against both electrical and chemical gradients is the result of excess OH^- in the cell after the H^+ has been pumped out.

The H^+,K^+-ATPase catalyzes the pumping of H^+ out of the cytoplasm into the secretory canaliculus in exchange for K^+. The exchange of H^+ for K^+ has a 1:1 stoichiometry and is therefore electrically neutral. In the resting cell, the H^+,K^+-ATPase is found in the membranes of the tubulovesicles. As noted previously, following a secretory stimulus, the tubulovesicles fuse with the canaliculus, thus greatly increasing the surface area of the secretory membrane and the number of "pumps" in it. When acid secretion ends, the tubulovesicles form again, and the canaliculus shrinks. Although there has been some controversy over whether the tubulovesicles are separate structures or whether they are collapsed canalicular membrane, current evidence indicates that they are separate structures that fuse with the canaliculus and undergo recycling following secretion. H^+,K^+-ATPase, like Na^+, K^+-ATPase, with which it has a 60% amino acid homology, is a member of the P-type ion-transporting ATPases, which also include the calcium (Ca^{2+})-ATPase. Inhibition of the H^+,K^+-ATPase totally blocks gastric acid secretion. Drugs such as omeprazole, a substituted benzimidazole, are accumulated in acid spaces and are activated at low pH. They then bind irreversibly to sulfhydryl groups of the H^+,K^+-ATPase and inactivate the enzyme. These pump inhibitors are the most potent of the different types of acid secretory inhibitors and are effective agents in the treatment of peptic ulcer, even ulcer caused by gastrinoma (Zollinger-Ellison syndrome).

ORIGIN OF THE ELECTRICAL POTENTIAL DIFFERENCE

The potential difference across the resting oxyntic gland mucosa is -70 to -80 millivolts (mV) lumen negative with respect to the blood. This charge separation is primarily caused by the secretion of Cl^- (see the previous section) against its electrochemical gradient. This is accomplished by both surface epithelial cells and parietal cells. Following the stimulation of acid secretion, the potential difference decreases to -30 or -40 mV because the positively charged H^+ moves in the same direction as Cl^-. H^+ therefore is actually secreted down its electrical gradient, thereby facilitating its transport against a several millionfold concentration gradient.

To produce an electrical gradient and a millionfold concentration gradient of H^+, there must be minimal leakage of ions and acid back into the mucosa. The ability of the stomach to prevent leakage is attributed to the so-called gastric mucosal barrier. If this barrier is disrupted by aspirin, alcohol, bile, or certain agents that damage the gastric mucosa, the potential difference decreases as ions leak down their electrochemical gradients. The exact nature of the barrier is unknown; its properties and the consequences of disrupting it are discussed more fully later, in the discussion of the pathophysiology of ulcer diseases. The negative potential difference across the stomach facilitates acid secretion because H^+ is secreted down the electrical gradient. The potential difference can be used to position catheters within the digestive tract. With an electrode placed at the catheter tip, the oxyntic gland mucosa can be distinguished readily from the esophagus (potential difference: -15 mV) or the duodenum (potential difference: -5 mV).

ELECTROLYTES OF GASTRIC JUICE

The concentrations of the major electrolytes in gastric juice are variable, but they are usually related to the rate of secretion (Fig. 8-5). At low rates the final juice is essentially a solution of NaCl with small amounts of H^+ and K^+. As the rate increases, the concentration of Na^+ decreases and that of H^+ increases. The concentrations of both Cl^- and K^+ rise slightly as the secretory rate rises. At peak rates, gastric juice is primarily HCl

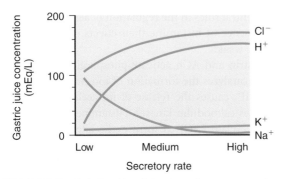

FIGURE 8-5 ■ Relationship of the electrolyte concentrations in gastric juice to the rate of gastric secretion. Cl⁻, chloride; H⁺, hydrogen ion; K⁺, potassium; Na⁺, sodium.

with small amounts of Na^+ and K^+. At all rates of secretion, the concentrations of H^+, K^+, and Cl^- are higher than those in plasma, and the concentration of Na^+ is lower than that in plasma. Thus gastric juice and plasma are approximately isotonic, regardless of the secretory rate.

To help understand the changes in ionic concentration, it is convenient to think of gastric juice as a mixture of two separate secretions: a nonparietal component and a parietal component. The nonparietal component is a basal alkaline secretion of constant and low volume. Its primary constituents are Na^+ and Cl^-, and it contains K^+ at about the same concentration as in plasma. In the absence of H^+ secretion, HCO_3^- can be detected in gastric juice. The HCO_3^- is secreted at a concentration of approximately 30 mEq/L. The nonparietal component is always present, and the parietal component is secreted against this background. As the rate of secretion increases, and because the increase is caused solely by the parietal component, the concentrations of electrolytes in the final juice begin to approach those of pure parietal cell secretion. Pure parietal cell secretion is slightly hyperosmotic and contains 150 to 160 mEq H^+/L and 10 to 20 mEq K^+/L. The only anion present is Cl^-.

This so-called two-component model of gastric secretion is an oversimplification. Parietal secretion is modified somewhat by the exchange of H^+ for Na^+ as the juice moves up the gland into the lumen. Although such changes are minimal, occurring primarily at low rates of secretion, they do participate in determining the final ionic composition of gastric juice.

Knowledge of the composition of gastric juice is required to treat a patient with chronic vomiting or one whose gastric juice is being aspirated and who is being maintained intravenously. Replacement of only NaCl and dextrose results in hypokalemic metabolic alkalosis, which can be fatal.

STIMULANTS OF ACID SECRETION

Only a few agents directly stimulate the parietal cells to secrete acid. The antral hormone gastrin and the parasympathetic mediator acetylcholine (ACh) are the most important physiologic regulators. ACh stimulates gastrin release in addition to stimulating the parietal cell directly.

Evidence has accumulated that an unknown hormone of intestinal origin also stimulates acid secretion. This substance tentatively has been named *entero-oxyntin* to denote both its origin and its action. In humans, circulating amino acids also stimulate the parietal cell and provide some of the stimulation of acid secretion that results from the presence of food in the small intestine.

Histamine, which occurs in many tissues (including the entire gastrointestinal [GI] tract), is a potent stimulator of parietal cell secretion. Histamine release is regulated by gastrin in most mammals, and it in turn stimulates acid secretion in the sense that gastrin and ACh do.

Role of Histamine in Acid Secretion

In 1920 Popielski, a Polish physiologist, discovered that histamine stimulated gastric acid secretion. It was then believed by many investigators that gastrin was actually histamine. The confusion cleared somewhat in 1938 when Komarov demonstrated two separate secretagogues in the gastric mucosa. He showed that trichloroacetic acid precipitated the peptide gastrin from gastric mucosal extracts, thus leaving histamine in the supernatant. MacIntosh then suggested that histamine was the final common mediator of acid secretion. He proposed that gastrin and ACh released histamine, which in turn stimulated the parietal cells directly and was the only direct stimulant of the parietal cells.

At this point it is important to introduce and define the concept of **potentiation.** Potentiation is said to occur between two stimulants if the response to their simultaneous administration exceeds the sum of the responses when each is administered alone. Certain secretory responses in the GI tract depend on the potentiation of two or more agonists. In the stomach histamine potentiates the effects of gastrin and ACh on the parietal cell. In this way small amounts of stimuli acting together can often produce a near-maximal secretory response. Potentiation requires the presence of separate receptors on the target cell for each stimulant and, in the case of acid secretion, is incompatible with the final common mediator hypothesis.

The first antihistamines discovered blocked only the histamine H_1 receptor, which mediates actions such as bronchoconstriction and vasodilation. The stimulation of acid secretion by histamine is mediated by the H_2 receptor and is not blocked by conventional antihistamines. The H_2 receptor antagonist **cimetidine** effectively inhibits histamine-stimulated acid secretion. Cimetidine, however, has also been found to inhibit the secretory responses to gastrin, ACh, and food. Atropine, a specific antagonist of the muscarinic actions of ACh, decreases the acid responses to gastrin and histamine as well as to ACh. When preparations of isolated parietal cells (which rule out the presence of stimuli other than those directly added) are used, investigators have shown that some effects of cimetidine on gastrin- and ACh-stimulated secretion are caused by inhibition of the part of the secretory response resulting from histamine potentiation. Similarly, the inhibition of gastrin- and histamine-stimulated secretion by atropine is caused by removal of the potentiating effects of ACh. Cimetidine is a more effective inhibitor of acid secretion than atropine and has fewer side effects. It is an extremely effective drug for the treatment of duodenal ulcer disease.

Histamine is found in **enterochromaffin-like** (ECL) **cells** within the lamina propria of the gastric glands. The relationships among gastrin, histamine, and ACh are shown in Figure 8-6. Located close to the parietal cells, ECL cells release histamine, which acts as a paracrine to stimulate acid secretion. ECL cells have cholecystokinin-2 (CCK-2) receptors for gastrin, which stimulate histamine release and synthesis and the growth of the ECL cells. ECL cells do not possess ACh receptors. The parietal cell membrane contains receptors for all three agonists. Parietal cells express histamine H_2 receptors, muscarinic M_3 receptors, and gastrin/CCK-2 receptors. Although gastrin and ACh

play central roles in the regulation of acid secretion, in the absence of histamine their effects on the parietal cell are weak.

Gastrin and ACh activate phospholipase C (PLC), which catalyzes the formation of inositol triphosphate (IP_3). IP_3 causes the release of intracellular Ca^{2+} and activates calmodulin kinases. Histamine activates adenylate cyclase (AC) to form cyclic adenosine monophosphate (cAMP), which activates protein kinase A. Protein kinase A and calmodulin kinases phosphorylate a variety of proteins to trigger the events leading to secretion and potentiate each other's effects. Thus the inhibition of acid secretion by histamine H_2 antagonists, such as cimetidine, results from both removal of potentiative interactions with histamine and inhibition of the stimulation caused by histamine released by gastrin.

STIMULATION OF ACID SECRETION

The unstimulated human stomach secretes acid at a rate equal to 10% to 15% of that present during

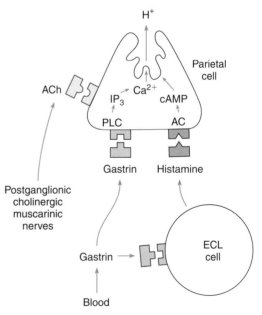

FIGURE 8-6 ■ The parietal cell contains receptors for gastrin, acetylcholine (ACh), and histamine. In addition, gastrin and ACh releases histamine from the enterochromaffin-like (ECL) cell. AC, adenylate cyclase; Ca^{2+}, calcium; cAMP, cyclic adenosine monophosphate; H^+, hydrogen ion; IP_3, inositol triphosphate; PLC, phospholipase C.

maximal stimulation. Basal acid secretion exhibits a diurnal rhythm with higher rates in the evening and lower rates in the morning before awakening. The cause of the diurnal variation is unknown because plasma gastrin is relatively constant during the interdigestive phase. The stomach emptied of food therefore contains a relatively small volume of gastric juice, and the pH of this fluid is usually less than 2. Thus in the absence of food the gastric mucosa is acidified.

The stimulation of gastric secretion is conveniently divided into three phases based on the location of the receptors initiating the secretory responses. This division is artificial; shortly after the start of a meal, stimulation is initiated from all three areas at the same time.

Cephalic Phase

Chemoreceptors and mechanoreceptors located in the tongue and the buccal and nasal cavities are stimulated by tasting, smelling, chewing, and swallowing food. The afferent nerve impulses are relayed through the vagal nucleus and vagal efferent fibers to the stomach. Even the thought or sight of an appetizing meal stimulates gastric secretion. The secretory response to cephalic stimulation depends greatly on the nature of the meal. The greatest response occurs to an appetizing self-selected meal. A bland meal produces a much smaller response. The efferent pathway for the cephalic phase is the vagus nerve. The entire response is blocked by vagotomy.

The cephalic phase is best studied by the procedure known as *sham feeding*. A dog is prepared with esophageal and gastric fistulas. When the esophageal fistula is open, swallowed food falls to the exterior without entering the stomach. Gastric secretion is collected from the gastric fistula, and its volume and acid content are measured. Stimulation during the cephalic phase represents approximately 30% of the total response to a meal. The cephalic phase also can be studied using a variety of drugs. Hypoglycemia introduced by tolbutamide or insulin, or interference with glucose metabolism by glucose analogues such as 3-methylglucose or 2-deoxyglucose, activates hypothalamic centers that stimulate secretion via the vagus nerve.

The vagus nerve acts directly on the parietal cells to stimulate acid secretion. It also acts on the antral gastrin cells (G cells) to stimulate gastrin release. The mediator at the parietal cells is ACh. The mediator at the gastrin cell is **gastrin-releasing peptide** (GRP) or **bombesin.** Within the antrum, postganglionic vagal neurons release both stimulatory and inhibitory neurotransmitters. Not all of these have been identified, and the overall response is the result of a complex process. The direct effect on the parietal cell is the more important in humans because selective vagotomy of the parietal cell–containing area of the stomach abolishes the response to sham feeding, whereas antrectomy only moderately reduces it. The mechanisms involved in the cephalic phase are illustrated in Figure 8-7.

Gastric Phase

Acid secretion during the gastric phase accounts for at least 50% of the response to a meal. When swallowed food first enters the stomach and mixes with the small volume of juice normally present, buffers (primarily protein) contained in the food neutralize the acid. The pH of the gastric contents may rise to 6 or more. Because gastrin release is inhibited when the antral pH drops below 3 and is prevented totally when the pH is

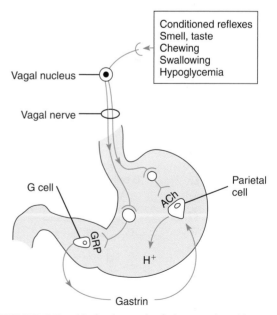

FIGURE 8-7 ■ Mechanisms stimulating gastric acid secretion during the cephalic phase. ACh, acetylcholine; G cell, gastrin-producing cell; GRP, gastrin-releasing peptide; H+, hydrogen ion.

less than 2, essentially no gastrin is released from a stomach that is void of food. The rise in pH permits vagal stimulation from the cephalic phase to initiate, and stimuli from the gastric phase to maintain, gastrin release. Increasing the pH of the gastric contents is not in itself a stimulus for gastrin release but merely allows other stimuli to be effective.

Distention of the stomach and bathing the gastric mucosa with certain chemicals, primarily amino acids, peptides, and amines, are the effective stimuli of the gastric phase. Distention activates mechanoreceptors in the mucosa of both the oxyntic and the pyloric gland areas initiating both long extramural reflexes and local, short intramural reflexes. All distention reflexes are mediated cholinergically and can be blocked by atropine.

Long reflexes also are called **vagovagal reflexes,** meaning that both afferent impulses and efferent impulses are carried by neurons in the vagus nerve. Mucosal distention receptors send signals by vagal afferents to the vagal nucleus. Efferent signals are sent back to G cells and parietal cells by the vagal efferents.

Short or local reflexes are mediated by neurons that are contained entirely within the wall of the stomach.

These may be single-neuron reflexes, or they may involve intermediary neurons. There are two local distention reflexes. Both are regional reflexes, meaning that the receptor and effector are located in the same area of the stomach. Distention of a vagally innervated pyloric (antrum) pouch stimulates gastrin release. The effect is decreased, but not abolished, by vagotomy, meaning that the gastrin response is mediated by both vagovagal reflexes and local reflexes. This local reflex is called a *pyloropyloric reflex.*

Distention of an antral pouch with pH 1 HCl stimulates acid secretion from the oxyntic gland area. Because gastrin release does not take place when the pH is below 2, the increase in acid output must be mediated by a neural reflex. As the discerning reader will have surmised, this vagovagal reflex is known as a *pyloro-oxyntic reflex.* Distention reflexes, which are much more effective stimulants of the parietal cell than they are of the G cell, are illustrated diagrammatically in Figure 8-8.

Peptides and amino acids stimulate gastrin release from the G cells. The most potent of these releasers are the aromatic amino acids. This effect is not blocked by

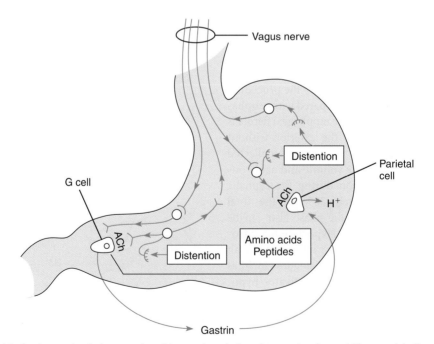

FIGURE 8-8 ■ Mechanisms stimulating gastric acid secretion during the gastric phase. ACh, acetylcholine; G cell, gastrin-producing cell; H+, hydrogen ion.

vagotomy. Only part of it appears to be blocked by atropine, a finding indicating that protein digestion products contain chemicals capable of directly stimulating the G cell to release gastrin. Acidification of the antral mucosa below pH 3 inhibits gastrin release in response to digested protein. A few other commonly ingested substances are also capable of stimulating acid secretion. Coffee, both caffeinated and decaffeinated, stimulates acid secretion. Ca^{2+}, either in the gastric lumen or as elevated serum concentrations, stimulates gastrin release and acid secretion. Considerable debate exists about the effects of alcohol on gastric secretion. Alcohol has been shown to stimulate gastrin release and acid secretion in some species; however, these effects do not seem to occur in humans.

Release of Gastrin

Considerable evidence has accumulated favoring the mechanism in Figure 8-9 to explain the regulation of gastrin release. GRP acts on the G cell to stimulate

gastrin release, and **somatostatin** acts on the G cell to inhibit release. GRP is a neurocrine released by vagal stimulation. This explains why atropine does not block vagally mediated gastrin release. Somatostatin acts as a paracrine, and its release is inhibited by vagal stimulation. In the isolated, perfused rat stomach, vagal stimulation increases GRP release and decreases somatostatin release into the perfusate. Thus vagal activation stimulates gastrin release by releasing GRP and inhibiting the release of somatostatin. Evidence also indicates that gastrin itself increases somatostatin release in a negative feedback manner.

Acid in the lumen of the stomach is believed to act directly on the somatostatin cell to stimulate the release of somatostatin, thereby preventing gastrin release. Protein digestion products—peptides, amino acids, and amines—may act directly on the G cell (or be absorbed by the G cell) to stimulate gastrin release. These substances most likely bind to receptors located on the apical membrane of the G cells, which are in contact with the gastric lumen.

Data indicate that atropine can block some gastrin release stimulated by protein digestion products. This is evidence that luminal receptors may be activated, resulting in a cholinergic reflex that leads to gastrin release. There is also evidence that this reflex may operate by releasing GRP and inhibiting somatostatin release.

Intestinal Phase

Protein digestion products in the duodenum stimulate acid secretion from denervated gastric mucosa, a finding indicating the presence of a hormonal mechanism. In humans, the proximal duodenum is rich in gastrin, which has been shown to contribute to the serum gastrin response to a meal. In dogs, liver extract releases a hormone from the duodenal mucosa that stimulates acid secretion without increasing serum gastrin levels. This hormone tentatively has been named *entero-oxyntin*. Its significance in humans is unknown.

Intravenous infusion of amino acids also stimulates acid secretion. Therefore a good portion of the stimulation attributed to the intestinal phase may be caused by absorbed amino acids. Intestinal stimuli result in only approximately 5% of the acid response to a meal. The gastric phase is responsible for most acid secretion.

Figure 8-10 summarizes the mechanisms and final stimulants acting in all three phases.

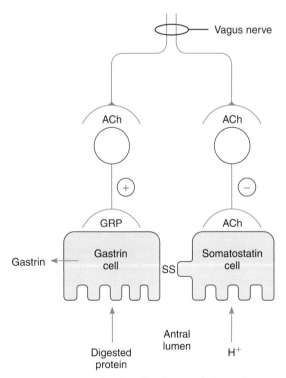

FIGURE 8-9 ■ Mechanism for the regulation of gastrin release. ACh, acetylcholine; GRP, gastrin-releasing peptide; H^+, hydrogen ion; SS, somatostatin.

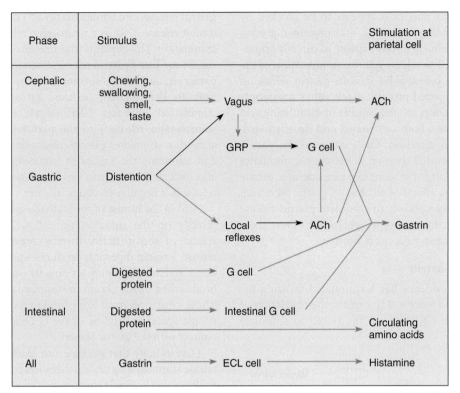

FIGURE 8-10 ■ Mechanisms for stimulating acid secretion. ACh, acetylcholine; ECL cell, enterochromaffin-like cell; G cell, gastrin-producing cell; GRP, gastrin-releasing peptide.

INHIBITION OF ACID SECRETION

When food first enters the stomach, its buffers neutralize the small volume of gastric acid present during the interdigestive phase. As the pH of the antral mucosa rises above 3, gastrin is released by the stimuli of the cephalic and gastric phases. One hour after the meal, the rate of gastric secretion is maximal, the buffering capacity of the meal is saturated, a significant portion of the meal has emptied from the stomach, and the acid concentration of the gastric contents increases. As the pH falls, gastrin release is inhibited, removing a significant factor for the stimulation of gastric acid secretion. This passive negative feedback mechanism is extremely important in the regulation of acid secretion. In addition, somatostatin released by the drop in intragastric pH also directly inhibits the parietal cells and inhibits the release of histamine from the ECL cells. The relationship between the rate of acid secretion and the pH and volume of the gastric contents is shown in Figure 8-11.

Evidence exists for several hormonal mechanisms for the inhibition of gastric acid secretion. These hormones are released from duodenal mucosa by acid, fatty acids, or hyperosmotic solutions and collectively are termed **enterogastrones.** They often inhibit gastric emptying as well as acid secretion. Teleologically these mechanisms ensure that the gastric contents are delivered to the small bowel at a rate that does not exceed the capacity for digestion and absorption. They also prevent damage to the duodenal mucosa that can result from acidic and hyperosmotic solutions.

Gastric inhibitory peptide (GIP) is released by fatty acids and acts at the parietal cell to inhibit acid secretion. **Secretin** may also be classified as an enterogastrone because it inhibits gastric acid secretion. The importance and physiologic significance of these effects in humans have not been determined.

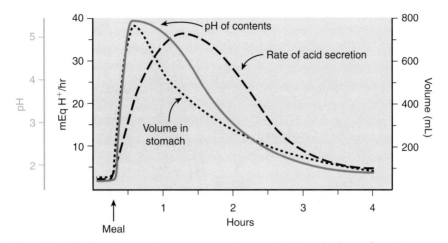

FIGURE 8-11 ■ The relationship between gastric secretory rate, intragastric pH, and volume of gastric contents during a meal. *(From Johnson LE: Essential Medical Physiology, 3rd ed. Philadelphia, Academic Press, 2003.)*

Region	Stimulus	Mediator	Inhibit gastrin release	Inhibit acid secretion
Oxyntic glands	Acid (pH <3.0)	Somatostatin		+
Antrum			+	
Duodenum	Acid	Secretin	+	+
		Nervous reflex		+
	Hyperosmotic solutions	Unidentified enterogastrone		+
Duodenum and jejunum	Fatty acids	GIP	+	+
		Unidentified enterogastrone		+

FIGURE 8-12 ■ Mechanisms for inhibiting acid secretion. GIP, gastric inhibitory peptide.

Cholecystokinin (CCK) is a physiologically significant inhibitor of gastric emptying. Hyperosmotic solutions release an as yet unidentified enterogastrone. Strong evidence also exists that acid initiates a nervous reflex from receptors in the duodenal mucosa that suppresses acid secretion. These mechanisms are summarized in Figure 8-12.

PEPSIN

Pepsinogen has a molecular weight of 42,500 and is split to form the active enzyme pepsin, which has a molecular weight of 35,000. Pepsinogen is converted to pepsin in the gastric juice when the pH drops below 5. Pepsin itself can catalyze the formation of additional pepsin

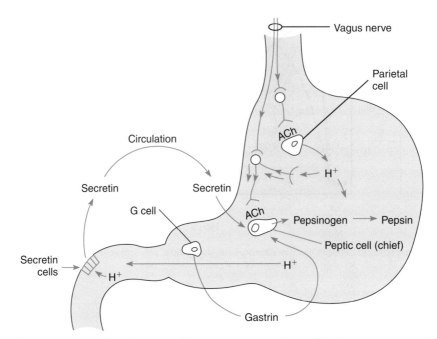

FIGURE 8-13 ■ Summary of mechanisms for stimulating pepsinogen secretion and activation to pepsin. ACh, acetylcholine; G cell, gastrin-producing cell; H$^+$, hydrogen ion.

from pepsinogen. Pepsin begins the digestion of protein by splitting interior peptide linkages (see Chapter 11).

Pepsinogens belong to two main groups: I and II. The pepsinogens in the first group are secreted by peptic and mucous cells of the oxyntic glands; those in the second group are secreted by mucous cells present in the pyloric gland area and duodenum, as well as in the oxyntic gland area. Pepsinogens appear in the blood, and considerable evidence indicates that their levels may be correlated with duodenal ulcer formation. This is discussed later in this chapter in connection with peptic ulcer disease.

The strongest stimulant of pepsinogen secretion is ACh. Thus vagal activation during both the cephalic and the gastric phases results in a significant proportion of the total pepsinogen secreted. H$^+$ plays an important role in several areas of pepsin physiology. First, acid is necessary to convert pepsinogen to the active enzyme pepsin. At pH 2 this conversion is almost instantaneous. Second, acid triggers a local cholinergic reflex that stimulates the chief cells to secrete. This mechanism is atropine sensitive and may account in part for the strong correlation between acid and pepsin outputs. Third, the acid-sensitive reflex

greatly enhances the effects of other stimuli on the peptic cell. This mechanism ensures that large amounts of pepsinogen are not secreted unless sufficient acid for conversion to pepsin is present. Fourth, acid releases the hormone secretin from duodenal mucosa. Secretin also stimulates pepsinogen secretion, although it is questionable whether enough secretin is present to do so under normal conditions.

The hormone gastrin is usually listed as a pepsigogue. The infusion of gastrin increases pepsin secretion. In dogs, the entire response can be accounted for by the stimulation of acid secretion by gastrin and the subsequent activation of the acid-sensitive reflex mechanism for pepsinogen secretion. In humans, gastrin may be a weak pepsigogue in its own right. The mechanisms regulating pepsinogen secretion are summarized in Figure 8-13.

Pepsin plays an important role in the ulceration of the stomach and duodenum, hence the term *peptic ulcer*. In the absence of pepsin, gastric acid does not produce an ulcer. Thus one of the benefits of the inhibition of acid secretion or neutralization of gastric acid during ulcer therapy may be the elimination of pepsin.

MUCUS

Vagal nerve stimulation and ACh increase soluble mucus secretion from the mucous neck cells. Soluble mucus consists of mucoproteins and mixes with the gastric chyme lubricating it.

Surface mucous cells secrete visible or insoluble mucus in response to chemical stimulants (e.g., ethanol) and in response to physical contact and friction with roughage in the diet. Visible mucus is secreted as a gel that entraps the alkaline component of the surface cell secretion. It is present during the interdigestive phase and protects the mucosa with an alkaline layer of lubricant. A portion of this coating is made up of mucus-containing surface cells that have been shed and trapped in the layer of mucus. During the response to a meal, insoluble mucus protects the mucosa from physical and chemical damage. It neutralizes a certain amount of acid and prevents pepsin from coming into contact with the mucosa. On contact with acid, insoluble mucus precipitates into clumps and passes into the duodenum with the chyme.

INTRINSIC FACTOR

Intrinsic factor is a mucoprotein with a molecular weight of 55,000 that is secreted by the parietal cells. It combines with vitamin B_{12} to form a complex that is necessary for the absorption of this vitamin by the ileal mucosa. Failure to secrete intrinsic factor is associated with achlorhydria and with the absence of parietal cells, which results in vitamin B_{12} deficiency or pernicious anemia. The development of this disease is poorly understood because the liver stores enough vitamin B_{12} to last several years. The condition is therefore not recognized until long after the changes have taken place in the gastric mucosa.

GROWTH OF THE MUCOSA

The growth of the GI mucosa is influenced by non-GI hormones and factors associated with the ingestion and digestion of a meal, such as GI hormones, nervous stimulation, secretions, and trophic substances present in the diet. Hypophysectomy results in atrophy of the digestive tract mucosa and the pancreas. The effects of hypophysectomy on growth can be prevented by administration of growth hormone. When administered to hypophysectomized rats, gastrin prevents atrophy of the GI mucosa and exocrine pancreas but does not affect the growth of other tissues. Interesting evidence indicates that adrenocortical steroids may trigger early postnatal development of the GI tract.

Gastrin is an important and necessary regulator of the growth of the oxyntic gland mucosa. It also stimulates growth of the intestinal and colonic mucosa and the exocrine pancreas. In humans, antrectomy causes atrophy of the remaining gastric mucosa; in rats, it causes atrophy of all GI mucosa (except that of the antrum and esophagus) and the exocrine pancreas. These changes are prevented by administration of exogenous gastrin. Hypergastrinemia results primarily in an increase in parietal and ECL cells. Gastrin is a potent stimulator of ECL cell proliferation via the CCK-2 receptor, and prolonged hypergastrinemia leads to ECL cell hyperplasia. Disruption of gastrin gene expression in mice inhibits parietal cell maturation and decreases their number. Conversely, overexpression of the gene results in increased proliferation of the gastric epithelium, increased number of parietal cells, and increased acid secretion.

Partial resection of the small intestine for tumor removal or for a variety of other reasons (e.g., treatment of morbid obesity) results in adaptation of the remaining mucosa. The mucosa of the entire digestive tract undergoes hyperplasia, which increases its ability to digest and transport nutrients or, in the case of the stomach, to secrete acid. Resection increases gastrin levels but not sufficiently to account for the adaptive changes. Evidence indicates that increased exposure of the mucosa to luminal contents plays an important role. After removal of proximal intestine, the distal intact mucosa is exposed to an increased load of pancreatic juice, bile, and nutrients. Investigators have hypothesized that bile and pancreatic juice contain growth factors that stimulate the adaptive response. The growth factors have not been isolated and tested. Increased uptake of nutrients by the distal mucosa has also been hypothesized to result in growth. The effects of specific nutrients have not been proved, and investigators disagree on whether growth is caused by an increased workload or an increase in the available supply of calories. Good evidence exists that a hormone different from gastrin also is involved in the adaptive response. This may be one of the glucagon-like peptides released from the distal small intestine.

The diet also contains polyamines that are required for growth. Trophic agents such as gastrin stimulate polyamine synthesis in the proliferative cells. Thus increased luminal polyamines from the diet, coupled with synthesis stimulated by trophic hormones, may explain some of the regulation of mucosal growth triggered by changes in the diet.

CLINICAL APPLICATIONS

Gastric and duodenal ulcers are lumped together under the heading of peptic ulcer disease. Although the formation of both types of ulcers requires acid and pepsin, their causes are basically different. Quite simply, an ulcer forms when damage from acid and pepsin overcomes the ability of the mucosa to protect itself and replace damaged cells. In the case of gastric ulcer, the defect is more often in the ability of the mucosa to withstand injury. In the case of duodenal ulcer, good evidence indicates that the mucosa is exposed to increased amounts of acid and pepsin. This analysis is an oversimplification because both factors are no doubt important in all cases of ulcer.

Representative acid secretory rates for normal individuals and for patients with gastrointestinal disorders are shown in Table 8-1. Maximal acid secretory output sometimes is measured but in itself is of little value in diagnosing ulcer disease. Normal subjects secrete approximately 25 mEq

TABLE 8-1

Comparison of Acid Output Values from the Human Stomach*

REPRESENTATIVE RANGES

Condition	Basal Acid Output (mEq/hr)	Maximal Acid Output (mEq/hr)
Normal	1-5	6-40
Gastric ulcer	0-3	1-20
Pernicious anemia	0	0-10
Duodenal ulcer	2-10	15-60
Zollinger-Ellison syndrome (gastrinoma)	10-30	30-80

*Basal acid output occurs at rest, and maximal acid output occurs during stimulation with histamine. The value is determined by multiplying the hourly volume of gastric juice aspirated times the hydrogen ion concentration of the juice.

hydrogen (H^+)/hour, in response to maximal injection of histamine, betazole, or gastrin. The mean output of patients with duodenal ulcer disease is approximately 40 mEq H^+/hour, but the degree of overlap among individuals is so great as to render the determination useless in diagnosis. The highest rates of acid secretion are seen in cases of gastrinoma (Zollinger-Ellison syndrome), but again individual overlap makes it impossible to differentiate between this condition and duodenal ulcer on the basis of secretory data alone. Lower than normal secretory rates are found in cases of gastric ulcer, and still lower secretory rates are found in patients with gastric carcinoma. Many patients in the latter two groups, however, fall well within the normal range.

Because of the feedback mechanism whereby antral acidification inhibits gastrin release, the general statement can be made that serum gastrin levels are related inversely to acid secretory capacity. Patients with gastric ulcer and carcinoma usually have higher than normal serum gastrin levels. Serum gastrin levels in pernicious anemia actually may approach those seen in gastrinoma. Obviously, patients with gastrinoma are an exception to this rule because their hypergastrinemia is derived not from the antrum but from a tumor not subject to inhibition by gastric acid. Except for the special tests mentioned in Chapter 1, serum gastrin levels cannot be used to differentiate various secretory abnormalities.

The decreased rate of acid secretion experienced with gastric ulcer is caused in part by the failure to recover acid that has been secreted and then has leaked back across the damaged gastric mucosa. The concept of the gastric mucosal

CLINICAL APPLICATIONS—cont'd

barrier is illustrated in Figure 8-14. The normal gastric mucosa is relatively impermeable to H^+. When the gastric mucosal barrier is weakened or damaged, H^+ leaks into the mucosa in exchange for sodium (Na^+). As H^+ accumulates in the mucosa, intracellular buffers are saturated, and the intracellular pH decreases, thus resulting in injury and cell death. Potassium (K^+) leaks from the damaged cells into the lumen. H^+ damages mucosal mast cells. They then release histamine, which exacerbates the condition by acting on H_1 receptors in the mucosal capillaries. The results are local ischemia, hypoxia, and vascular stasis. Plasma proteins and pepsin leak into the gastric juice; if damage is severe, bleeding will occur. Common agents that produce mucosal damage of this type are aspirin, ethanol, and bile salts. The mucosal lesions produced by topical damage to the gastric barrier may be forerunners of gastric ulcer.

The exact nature of the barrier is unknown. It is probably physiologic as well as anatomic. Cell membranes and junctional complexes prevent normal back-diffusion of H^+. Diffused H^+ normally is transported actively back into the lumen. Factors that have been speculated to play a role in maintaining mucosal resistance are blood flow, mucus, bicarbonate secretion, cellular renewal, and chemical factors such as gastrin, prostaglandins, and epidermal growth factor. The last three agents

have all been shown to decrease the severity and promote the healing of gastric ulcers.

Factors that have been elucidated as important in duodenal ulcer formation pertain to acid and pepsin secretion. Patients with duodenal ulcer have on the average 2 billion parietal cells and can secrete approximately 40 mEq H^+/hour. Comparable measurements for normal individuals are approximately 50% of this number. In addition, the secretion of pepsin is doubled in the duodenal ulcer group, as can be detected by measuring plasma pepsinogen. Although fasting serum gastrin is normal in patients with duodenal ulcer, the gastrin response to a meal and sensitivity to gastrin are increased. Increased serum gastrin after a meal is caused in part by the fact that acid suppresses gastrin release less effectively in patients with duodenal ulcer than in controls. The increased parietal cell mass may therefore be caused by the trophic effect of gastrin.

The major acquired factor in the origin of both gastric ulcer and duodenal ulcer is the bacterium *Helicobacter pylori*. The infection is found in 80% of patients with duodenal ulcer and virtually 100% of patients with gastric ulcers whose ulcers were not caused by the long-term use of aspirin or other nonsteroidal anti-inflammatory drugs (NSAIDs). *H. pylori* is a gram-negative bacterium, characterized by high urease activity, which metabolizes

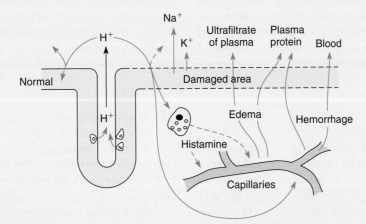

FIGURE 8-14 ■ Events that follow damage to the gastric mucosal barrier. H^+, hydrogen ion; K^+, potassium; Na^+, sodium.

Continued

urea into ammonia to neutralize gastric acid. This reaction allows the bacterium to withstand the acid environment of the stomach and to colonize the mucosa. The resulting production of ammonium (NH_4^+) is believed to be a major cause of cytotoxicity because NH_4^+ directly damages epithelial cells and increases the permeability of the mucosa (i.e., it "breaks the mucosal barrier"). The bacteria produce numerous other factors, such as platelet-activating factor and cytokines, that also damage cells. All these factors probably contribute to gastric ulcer formation. *H. pylori* infection can progress from gastritis to gastric cancer.

NSAIDs inhibit the enzyme cyclooxygenase, thereby reducing the synthesis of prostaglandins (PGE_2 and PGI_2) from arachidonic acid. The prostaglandins are normally protective, and the increased arachidonic acid results in the production of leukotriene B_4 (LTB_4) and subsequent neutrophil adhesion to the walls of mucosal capillaries. This process leads to ischemia and mucosal damage.

H. pylori also causes the increased acid secretion associated with duodenal ulcer. Compared with normal individuals, patients with duodenal ulcer have increased basal acid output, increased gastrin-releasing peptide (GRP)-stimulated acid output, increased maximal acid output in response to gastrin, increased ratio of basal acid output to gastrin-stimulated maximal acid output, and increased ratio of GRP-stimulated maximal acid output to gastrin-stimulated maximal acid output. All these findings, except the increased maximal acid output in response to gastrin, totally disappeared following eradication of the *H. pylori* infection. The increased acid secretory and serum gastrin responses to GRP appear to be related to a decreased inhibition of gastrin release and parietal cell secretion by somatostatin in *H. pylori*–infected persons. Patterns of *H. pylori*–related gastritis differ in gastric and duodenal ulcer. Gastric ulcers are associated with diffuse gastritis, whereas duodenal ulcers are associated predominantly with the infection of the antrum. Although all the mechanisms by which *H. pylori* affects the mucosa have not been elucidated, the information available coincides with the known pathophysiology of both gastric and duodenal ulcer diseases.

Medical treatment of duodenal ulcer disease usually consists of administering antacids to neutralize secreted acid or a histamine H_2-receptor blocker to inhibit secretion. The H^+,K^+-ATPase (proton pump) inhibitor omeprazole blocks all acid secretion. It is extremely effective in treating duodenal ulcers, even those caused by gastrinoma. Surgical treatment is based entirely on physiology. The most commonly used operations are vagotomy and antrectomy. These procedures result in a 60% to 70% decrease in acid secretion by removing one or both major stimulants of acid secretion. With the advent of the H_2 blockers and proton pump inhibitors, ulcers are now rarely treated by surgical intervention. To prevent recurrence, physicians eradicate *H. pylori*. This is best done by giving antibiotics in combination with omeprazole, which increases the susceptibility of the bacteria to antibiotic treatment.

SUMMARY

1. The functions of gastric juice are attributed to acid, pepsin, intrinsic factor, mucus, and water.

2. Acid is secreted in concentrations as high as 150 mEq/L at high rates of secretion; the acid converts inactive pepsinogen to the active enzyme pepsin, kills bacteria, and solubilizes some foodstuffs.

3. Acid is secreted by the parietal cells, which contain the enzyme H^+,K^+-ATPase on their apical secretory membranes.

4. The concentrations of the electrolytes in gastric juice vary with the rate of secretion.

5. The three major stimulants of acid secretion are the hormone gastrin, the cholinergic neuromediator ACh, and the paracrine histamine, which is released from ECL cells in response to gastrin.

6. During the cephalic phase of secretion, vagal activation stimulates the parietal cells directly via ACh and releases gastrin from the G cells via GRP.

7. During the gastric phase of secretion, distention of the wall of the stomach stimulates the parietal cells and releases gastrin via both mucosal and vagovagal reflexes; protein digestion products stimulate the G cells directly to release gastrin.

8. When the pH of luminal contents drops below 3, somatostatin is released from D cells in the antrum and oxyntic gland area, where it inhibits gastrin release, histamine release from ECL cells, and acid secretion.

9. Acid secretion is inhibited further when chyme enters the duodenum, triggers the release of inhibitory hormones, and initiates inhibitory neural reflexes.

10. Pepsinogen secretion is stimulated by vagal activation and ACh and by acid in the lumen of the stomach.

11. Intrinsic factor, secreted by the parietal cells, is required for the absorption of vitamin B_{12} by a specific carrier mechanism located in the ileum.

KEY WORDS AND CONCEPTS

Intrinsic factor

Hydrogen ion

Pepsin

Mucus

Water

Gastric mucosal barrier

Oxyntic gland area

Pyloric gland area

Antrum

Parietal cells

Peptic/chief cells

Pepsinogen

Tubulovesicles

Intracellular canaliculus

Carbonic anhydrase

H^+,K^+-ATPase

Histamine

Potentiation

Cimetidine

Enterochromaffin-like cells

Gastrin-releasing peptide/ bombesin

Vagovagal reflexes

Somatostatin

Enterogastrones

Gastric inhibitory peptide

Secretin

Cholecystokinin

SUGGESTED READINGS

Beaumont W: *Experiments and Observations on the Gastric Juice and the Physiology of Digestion*, New York, 1955, Dover.

Chan FK, Leung WK: Peptic ulcer disease, *Lancet* 360:933–940, 2002.

El-Omar EM, Penman ID, Ardill JES, et al: *Helicobacter pylori* infection and abnormalities of acid secretion in patients with duodenal ulcer disease, *Gastroenterology* 109:681–691, 1995.

Feldman M, Richardson CT: Gastric acid secretion in humans. In Johnson LR, editor: *Physiology of the Gastrointestinal Tract*, vol 1, New York, 1981, Raven Press.

Okamot C, Karvar S, Forte JG, Yao X: The cell biology of gastric acid secretion. In Johnson LR, editor: ed 5, *Physiology of the Gastrointestinal Tract*, vol 2, San Diego, 2012, Elsevier.

Hersey SJ: Gastric secretion of pepsinogen. In Johnson LR, editor: ed 3, *Physiology of the Gastrointestinal Tract*, vol 2, New York, 1994, Raven Press.

Johnson LR, McCormack SA: Regulation of gastrointestinal growth. In Johnson LR, editor: ed 3, *Physiology of the Gastrointestinal Tract*, vol 1, New York, 1994, Raven Press.

Lindström E, Chen D, Norlen P, et al: Control of gastric acid secretion: the gastrin–ECL cell–parietal cell axis, *Comp Biochem Physiol A Mol Integr Physiol* 128:505–514, 2001.

Modlin IM, Sachs G: *Acid Related Diseases*, Milan, 1998, Schnetztor-Verlag Gmbh D-Konstanz.

Polk DB, Frey MR: Mucosal restitution and repair. In Johnson LR, editor: ed 5, *Physiology of the Gastrointestinal Tract*, vol 1, 2012, San Diego, Elsevier.

Schubert ML: Regulation of gastric acid secretion. In Johnson LR, editor: ed 5, *Physiology of the Gastrointestinal Tract*, vol 2, San Diego, 2012, Elsevier.

Silen W: Gastric mucosal defense and repair. In Johnson LR, editor: ed 2, *Physiology of the Gastrointestinal Tract*, vol 2, New York, 1987, Raven Press.

PANCREATIC SECRETION

OBJECTIVES

- Describe the two components of pancreatic exocrine secretion, their cells of origin, and their functions.
- Understand the mechanisms involved in the formation of both the electrolyte (aqueous) and enzymatic components of pancreatic secretion.
- Explain the hormonal and neural regulation of both the aqueous and enzymatic components of pancreatic secretion.
- Discuss the cellular basis for potentiation and its importance in the pancreatic response to a meal.
- Discuss the various clinical conditions resulting from the decreased production of either or both the aqueous and enzymatic components of pancreatic juice.
- Understand how the preceding clinical conditions may arise.

Pancreatic exocrine secretion is divided conveniently into an aqueous or bicarbonate (HCO_3^-) component and an enzymatic component. The function of the **aqueous component** is the neutralization of the duodenal contents. As such, it prevents damage to the duodenal mucosa by acid and pepsin and brings the pH of the contents into the optimal range for activity of the pancreatic enzymes. The **enzymatic** or **protein component** is a low-volume secretion containing enzymes for the digestion of all normal constituents of a meal. Unlike the enzymes secreted by the stomach and salivary glands, the pancreatic enzymes are essential to normal digestion and absorption.

FUNCTIONAL ANATOMY

The exocrine pancreas can best be likened to a cluster of grapes, and its functional units resemble the salivons of the salivary glands. Groups of acini form lobules separated by areolar tissue. Each acinus is formed from several pyramidal **acinar cells** oriented with their apices toward the lumen. The lumen of the spherical acinus is drained by a ductule whose epithelium extends into the acinus in the form of centroacinar cells. Ductules join to form intralobular ducts, which in turn drain into interlobular ducts. These join the major pancreatic duct draining the gland.

The acinar cells secrete a small volume of juice rich in protein. Essentially all the proteins present in pancreatic juice are digestive enzymes. **Ductule cells** and **centroacinar cells** produce a large volume of watery secretion containing sodium (Na^+) and HCO_3^- as its major constituents.

Distributed throughout the pancreatic parenchyma are the **islets of Langerhans** or the endocrine pancreas. The islets produce insulin from the beta cells and glucagon from the alpha cells. In addition, the pancreas produces the candidate hormone pancreatic polypeptide and contains large amounts of somatostatin, which may act as a paracrine to inhibit the release of insulin and glucagon.

The efferent nerve supply to the pancreas includes both sympathetic and parasympathetic nerves. Sympathetic postganglionic fibers emanate from the celiac and superior mesenteric plexuses and accompany the arteries to the organ. Parasympathetic preganglionic fibers are distributed by branches of the vagi coursing down the antral-duodenal region. Hence, surgical vagotomy for peptic ulcer disease affects not only the intended target organ, the hypersecreting stomach, but also the pancreas. More recently, more selective operations have been designed to resect only the vagal branches passing to the stomach. Vagal fibers terminate either at acini and islets or at the intrinsic cholinergic nerves of the pancreas. In general, the sympathetic nerves inhibit, and the parasympathetic nerves stimulate, pancreatic exocrine secretion.

MECHANISMS OF FLUID AND ELECTROLYTE SECRETION

The pancreas secretes approximately 1 L of fluid per day. At all rates of secretion, pancreatic juice is essentially isotonic with extracellular fluid. At low rates the primary ions are Na^+ and chloride (Cl^-). At high rates Na^+ and HCO_3^- predominate. Potassium ions (K^+) are present at all rates of secretion at a concentration equal to their concentration in plasma. The concentrations of Na^+ in pancreatic juice and in plasma also are approximately equal.

The aqueous component is secreted by the ductule and centroacinar cells and may contain 120 to 140 milliequivalents (mEq) of HCO_3^-/L, several times its concentration in plasma. The electropotential difference across the ductule epithelium is 5 to 9 millivolts (mV), lumen negative. Hence HCO_3^- is secreted against both electrical and chemical gradients. This is often considered evidence that HCO_3^- is transported actively across the luminal surface of the cells. Although the exact mechanism involved in pancreatic HCO_3^- secretion is unknown, the current model is shown in Figure 9-1. This model is based on information that shows the following: (1) more than 90% of HCO_3^- in pancreatic juice is derived from plasma; (2) the secretion of HCO_3^- occurs against an electrochemical gradient and is an active process; (3) HCO_3^- secretion is blocked by ouabain, meaning that Na^+,K^+-adenosine triphosphatase (ATPase) is involved; (4) HCO_3^- secretion involves Na^+-hydrogen ion (H^+) and Cl^--HCO_3^- exchangers and carbonic anhydrase; and (5) HCO_3^- secretion is decreased significantly in the absence of extracellular Cl^-. In Figure 9-1, most of the HCO_3^- enters the cell across the basolateral membrane cotransported with

Na^+. Intracellular HCO_3^- is also produced by the diffusion of carbon dioxide (CO_2) into the cell, its hydration by carbonic anhydrase, and dissociation into H^+ and HCO_3^-. The H^+ is transported across the basolateral membrane by the Na^+-H^+ exchanger. Both these steps depend on the Na^+ gradient established by Na^+,K^+-ATPase. When H^+ reaches the plasma, it combines with HCO_3^- to produce additional CO_2. In some species such as the rat, HCO_3^- enters the lumen in exchange for Cl^-.

In humans and other species able to secrete HCO_3^- in concentrations up to 140 mEq/L, HCO_3^- enters through a channel that is also able to secrete Cl^-. The rate of HCO_3^- secretion depends on the availability of luminal Cl^-, which is dependent on the opening of this channel in the apical membrane. This channel, which is the cystic fibrosis transmembrane conductance regulator (CFTR), is activated by cyclic adenosine monophosphate (cAMP) in response to stimulation by secretin and is present in duct cells but not acinar cells. Na^+ moves paracellularly down the established electrochemical gradient from the plasma to the lumen of the gland. Water passively moves from the plasma into the lumen, down the osmotic gradient created by the secretion of Na^+ and HCO_3^-. Most water moves through aquaporin 1 channels in both the basolateral and apical membranes. This secretion is similar to that occurring in the parietal cells of the stomach, except that the H^+ and HCO_3^- are transported in opposite directions. Thus the venous blood from an actively secreting pancreas has a lower pH than that from an inactive gland.

As in gastric juice, the ionic concentrations in pancreatic juice vary with the rate of secretion (Fig. 9-2). The concentrations of anions (Cl^- and HCO_3^-) in pancreatic juice are related inversely to each other, as are the concentrations of cations (Na^+ and H^+) in gastric juice. Because these relationships are analogous, it may be surmised that analogous theories have been proposed to explain them:

■ The two-component hypothesis assumes that one cell type, the acinar cell, secretes a small amount of fluid whose major ions are Na^+ and Cl^-. The duct cells secrete large volumes of juice rich in Na^+ and HCO_3^- in response to stimulation. At low rates of secretion, the Cl^- concentration of

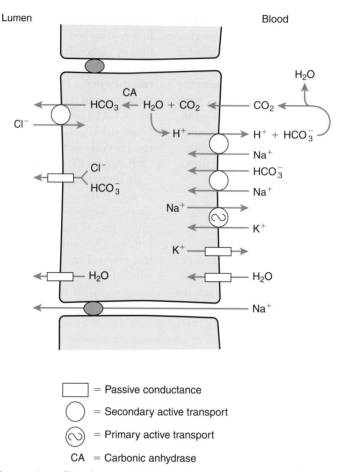

Lumen   Blood

FIGURE 9-1 ▧ Model for the secretion of bicarbonate (HCO_3^-) by the pancreatic duct cell. Cl^-, chloride; CO_2, carbon dioxide; H^+, hydrogen ion; H_2O, water; K^+, potassium; Na^+, sodium.

the juice is therefore relatively high. As the secretory rate increases, the fixed amount of Cl^- being secreted is diluted by the much larger volume of HCO_3^--containing juice, and the final concentrations of the two anions approach those in the pure HCO_3^- secretion.

- Another theory proposes that the cells primarily secrete HCO_3^- and that, as it moves down the ducts, it is exchanged for Cl^-. At low rates of secretion, there is sufficient time for the exchange to be nearly complete, and the concentration of each anion is equal to its concentration in plasma. As the rate of secretion increases, less time is available for exchange, and the final ionic makeup of pancreatic juice approaches that of

the originally secreted solution containing only HCO_3^- and Na^+.

Both processes probably are involved in determining the final composition of the secreted juice.

MECHANISMS OF ENZYME SECRETION

The exocrine pancreas has the highest daily rate of protein synthesis of any organ in the body. A liter of pancreatic juice may contain 10 to 100 g of protein that enters the intestine each day. The pancreatic acinar cells synthesize and secrete major enzymes for the digestion of all three primary foodstuffs. Like pepsin,

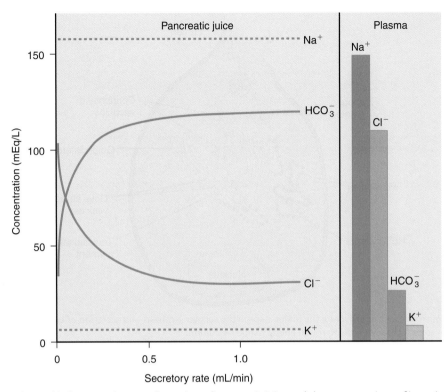

FIGURE 9-2 ▪ Relationship between the rate of secretion of pancreatic juice and the concentrations of its major ions. Cl⁻, chloride; HCO₃⁻, bicarbonate; K⁺, potassium; Na⁺, sodium.

the pancreatic proteases are secreted as inactive enzyme precursors and are converted to active forms in the lumen. Pancreatic amylase and lipase are secreted in active forms. The activation and specific actions of the pancreatic enzymes are covered in detail in Chapter 11.

Although a certain amount of controversy exists concerning the mechanisms of the synthesis and secretion of enzymes by the acinar cells, the process outlined in Figure 9-3 is accepted by most authorities. The secretory process begins with the synthesis of exportable proteins in association with polysomes attached to the cisternae of the rough endoplasmic reticulum (RER) (step 1). As it is being synthesized, the elongating protein, directed by a leader sequence of hydrophobic amino acids, enters the cisternal cavity, where it is collected after synthesis is complete (step 2).

Once within the cisternal space, enzymes remain membrane bound until they are secreted from the cell. The enzymes next move through the cisternae of the

RER to transitional elements, which are associated with smooth vesicles at the Golgi periphery. Possibly as a result of pinching off the transitional elements containing them, the enzymes become associated with the Golgi vesicles (step 3), which transport them to condensing vacuoles (step 4). Energy is required for transport through the endoplasmic reticulum and Golgi vesicles to the condensing vacuoles. Within the condensing vacuoles, the enzymes are concentrated to form zymogen granules (step 5). They are then stored in the zymogen granules that collect at the apex of the cell. After a secretory stimulus, the membrane of the zymogen granule fuses with the cell membrane, thus ultimately rupturing and expelling the enzymes into the lumen (step 6). This is the only step in the process that requires a secretory stimulus. The human acinar cell does not have cholecystokinin 1 (CCK1) receptors, so CCK does not stimulate secretion directly. CCK activates cholinergic reflexes via CCK1 receptors, and acetylcholine (Ach) activates muscarinic receptors on

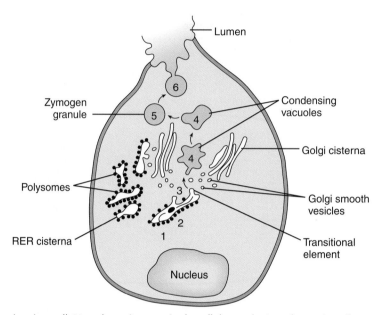

FIGURE 9-3 ■ Pancreatic acinar cell. Note the major steps in the cellular synthesis and secretion of enzymes, and see the text for an explanation of steps 1 through 6. RER, rough endoplasmic reticulum.

the acinar cell. The results are a release of calcium (Ca^{2+}) from the endoplasmic reticulum and the subsequent activation of protein kinases, which stimulate exocytosis.

REGULATION OF SECRETION

As may be expected from its function to neutralize the duodenum, the secretion of fluid and HCO_3^- (the aqueous component) is largely determined by the amount of acid entering the duodenum. The secretion of pancreatic enzymes is similarly determined primarily by the amount of fat and protein entering the duodenum. Control of pancreatic secretion is regulated primarily by secretin, CCK, and vagovagal reflexes. Intestinal stimuli account for most pancreatic secretion, but secretion is also stimulated during the cephalic and gastric phases.

Basal pancreatic secretion in humans is low and difficult to measure. The basal secretion of HCO_3^- is 2% to 3% of maximal, and basal enzyme secretion is 10% to 15% of maximal. The stimuli for basal secretion are unknown. Because the isolated perfused pancreas secretes basally, this secretion may be an intrinsic property of the gland.

Cephalic Phase

Truncal vagotomy reduces the pancreatic secretory response to a meal by approximately 60%. Most of this decrease is caused by the interruption of vagovagal reflexes and the removal of the potentiating and sensitizing effects of ACh that increase the response to secretin. However, a direct vagal component of stimulation is initiated during the cephalic phase. Sham feeding produces a pancreatic secretory response that, of course, is blocked totally by vagotomy. In dogs, the cephalic phase accounts for approximately 20% of the response to a meal. The stimuli for the cephalic phase of pancreatic secretion are the conditioned reflexes, smell, taste, chewing, and swallowing. Afferent impulses travel to the vagal nucleus. Vagal efferents to the pancreas stimulate both the ductule and the acinar cells to secrete. Stimulation is mediated by ACh and has a greater effect on the enzymatic component than it does on the aqueous component. In dogs, a portion of the cephalic phase is mediated by gastrin released by the vagus. Gastrin has approximately half the potency of CCK for activating the acinar cells. Gastrin plays only a minor role, if any, in the regulation of human pancreatic secretion. These mechanisms are illustrated in Figure 9-4.

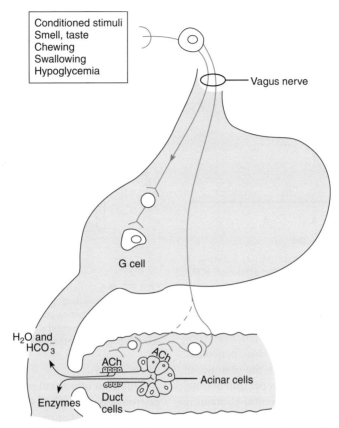

FIGURE 9-4 ▨ Mechanisms involved in the stimulation of pancreatic secretion during the cephalic phase. *Dashed lines* represent minor effects. ACh, acetylcholine; HCO_3^-, bicarbonate; H_2O, water.

Gastric Phase

The stimulation of pancreatic secretion originating from food in the stomach is mediated by the same mechanisms that are involved in the cephalic phase. Distention of the wall of the stomach initiates vagovagal reflexes to the pancreas. Gastrin is released by protein digestion products and distention (see Chapter 8), but again it plays little or no role in the stimulation of the human pancreas.

Intestinal Phase

The presence of digestion products and H^+ in the human small intestine accounts for 70% to 80% of the stimulation of pancreatic secretion. Secretin and CCK account for almost all the hormonal stimulation of pancreatic secretion. The stimulus for the alkaline component (water and HCO_3^-) is secretin released from the S cells by gastric acid and high concentrations of long-chain fatty acids. Secretion of the enzymatic component from the acinar cells is stimulated by CCK released from the I cells by fat and protein digestion products. Current evidence indicates that human acinar cells lack CCK receptors. Because vagotomy blocks the secretory response to infusions of physiologic doses of CCK, in humans, CCK acts by stimulating vagal afferent receptors and initiating vagovagal reflexes. This stimulation depends on cholinergic signaling because atropine blocks pancreatic secretion in response to CCK. In rodents, acinar cells express CCK receptors and are activated directly by the hormone.

The only potent releaser of secretin is H^+. The duodenal pH threshold for secretin release is 4.5. Secretin release rises almost linearly as the pH is lowered to 3 (Fig. 9-5). Lowering the pH below 3 does not lead to

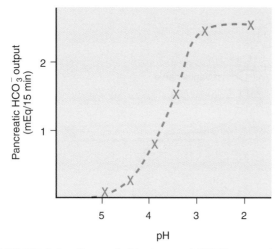

FIGURE 9-5 ■ Pancreatic bicarbonate (HCO_3^-) output in response to various duodenal pH values. The output of HCO_3^- is used as an index of secretin release.

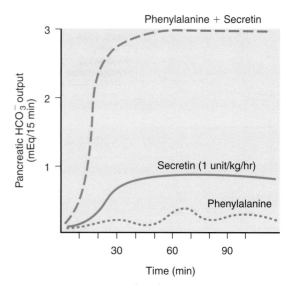

FIGURE 9-6 ■ Pancreatic bicarbonate (HCO_3^-) output in response to continual perfusion of the duodenum with phenylalanine, to continuous intravenous infusion of secretin, and to the combination of the two stimuli. The response to secretin is greatly potentiated by endogenous phenylalanine.

greater release of secretin, provided the amount of titratable acid entering the duodenum is held constant. Below pH 3, secretin release and pancreatic HCO_3^- secretion are related only to the amount of titratable acid entering the duodenum per unit of time. As more acid enters the gut, more secretin-containing cells are stimulated to release hormone. Thus at a constant pH, the amount of secretin released is a function of the length of gut acidified. Secretin can be released from the entire duodenum and jejunum, and the amount of hormone available for release appears to be constant per centimeter of proximal small intestine.

During the response to a normal meal, however, only the duodenal bulb and proximal duodenum are acidified sufficiently to release secretin. The pH of the proximal duodenum rarely drops below 4 to 3.5. This finding raises doubts about whether sufficient secretin is released by a meal to account for the high rates of pancreatic HCO_3^- and water secretion normally seen. If the pH of the gastric contents entering the duodenum is kept at 5 or higher by automatic titration, the pancreatic response is typical of CCK and ACh acting alone (a small volume of enzyme-rich juice). Dropping the pH even slightly below the threshold for secretin release leads to large increases in volume and HCO_3^- secretion. The conclusion therefore is that the effects of a small amount of secretin are potentiated by CCK and ACh. In humans, this potentiation is the result of ACh alone.

This is an important physiologic interaction of two gastrointestinal (GI) hormones and cholinergic reflexes and is demonstrated directly by the experiment outlined in Figure 9-6. Phenylalanine, a potent releaser of CCK and initiator of vagovagal reflexes, produces a small increase in volume when given alone. If, however, the same dose is infused into the gut while a low dose of secretin is given intravenously, the output of the pancreatic alkaline component increases to levels seen during a meal. Vagotomy greatly decreases the potentiated response. Physiologically, then, in humans, the volume and HCO_3^- responses to a meal result from small amounts of secretin released by duodenal acidification, potentiated by ACh from vagovagal reflexes activated by CCK.

Secretin has been referred to as "nature's antacid" because most of its physiologic and pharmacologic actions decrease the amount of acid in the duodenum. For example, it stimulates secretion of HCO_3^- from the pancreas and liver and inhibits gastric secretion and emptying, as well as gastrin release.

CCK is the principal humoral regulator of enzyme secretion from the pancreatic acinar cells. It is released in response to amino acids and fatty acids in the small intestine. Only L-isomers of amino acids are effective. In dogs, phenylalanine and tryptophan are potent releasers. Alanine, leucine, and valine are less effective. Phenylalanine, methionine, and valine appear to be potent releasers in humans. CCK is distributed evenly over the first 90 cm of intestine, and infusion of L-phenylalanine below the ligament of Treitz produces pancreatic enzyme responses equal to those seen after infusion near the pylorus. Thus the amount of CCK released depends on the load and length of bowel exposed, as well as on the concentration of amino acids present.

Strong evidence indicates that some peptides, as well as single amino acids, also release CCK. Three dipeptides, all of which contain glycine (*glycylphenylalanine, glycyltryptophan,* and *phenylalanylglycine),* are effective. Dipeptides or tripeptides of glycine, or glycine itself, are ineffective. Evidence exists that some peptides containing at least four amino acids are also effective. Undigested protein does not release CCK. After a protein meal, therefore, many different specific protein products evoke CCK release and pancreatic enzyme secretion.

In addition to protein products, fatty acids longer than eight carbon atoms release CCK and initiate vagovagal reflexes. *Lauric, palmitic, stearic,* and *oleic acids* are equal and strong releasers of CCK. Fat must be in an absorbable form before release of the hormone occurs. The interactions between luminal nutrients and the receptors triggering the release of CCK, and of GI hormones in general, are poorly understood. As a result, most of the intracellular mechanisms resulting in hormone release are unknown. Part of the reason for this paucity of information has been the inability to isolate large numbers of hormone-containing cells from the mucosa of the GI tract.

Active trypsin in the intestinal lumen inhibits CCK release, and the ingestion of trypsin inhibitors strongly stimulates the release of the hormone. Diversion of pancreatic secretion from the gut lumen also increases plasma CCK. These data suggest the existence of a feedback mechanism controlling the release of CCK. Additional studies indicate that dietary protein products bind or inhibit trypsin, which would otherwise inactivate a CCK-releasing peptide. Several of these peptides have been identified, but their physiologic significance remains to be elucidated.

The mechanisms resulting in the stimulation of pancreatic secretion during the intestinal phase are illustrated in Figure 9-7.

CELLULAR BASIS FOR POTENTIATION

The concept of **potentiation** requires that the potentiating stimuli act on different membrane receptors and trigger different cellular mechanisms for the stimulation of secretion. Some of the steps in these mechanisms have been elucidated for the rodent pancreatic acinar cell; these are illustrated in Figure 9-8.

Secretin binding to its receptor triggers an increase in adenylyl cyclase activity that results in the synthesis of cAMP. ACh and CCK bind to separate receptors, but both increase intracellular Ca^{2+}. The Ca^{2+} is mobilized primarily from the plasma membranes and RER of the acinar cells. Both CCK and ACh also increase diacylglycerol and inositol triphosphate (IP_3) production from phosphatidylinositol. It is likely that one of these breakdown products is the intracellular messenger for Ca^{2+} release. Interactions between secretin and ACh or secretin and CCK result in potentiation. However, the effects of combining CCK and ACh, which trigger identical mechanisms, are only additive. Glucagon and vasoactive intestinal peptide (VIP) also increase cAMP. Gastrin, gastrin-releasing peptide, and substance P increase Ca^{2+} in acinar cells. However, no strong evidence indicates that these substances play an important role in the physiologic regulation of pancreatic secretion.

The final steps in the process leading to enzyme secretion have not been elucidated, but they involve the phosphorylation of structural and regulatory proteins. Potentiation occurs because Ca^{2+} and cAMP lead to the activation of different kinases and the phosphorylation of different proteins. The foregoing interactions have been worked out with guinea pig isolated pancreatic acini. Secretin does not potentiate the effects of CCK and ACh in dogs or humans. A system similar to this, however, is a likely explanation of the potentiation in all species in which it occurs. Thus similar events may be predicted for the human ductule cell, in which secretin (cAMP) is potentiated by ACh (Ca^{2+}).

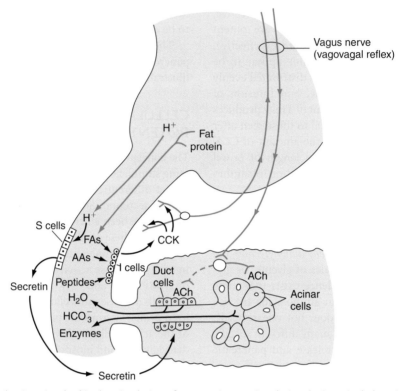

FIGURE 9-7 ■ Mechanisms involved in the stimulation of pancreatic secretion during the intestinal phase in the human. *Dashed lines* indicate potentiative interactions. AAs, amino acids; ACh, acetylcholine; CCK, cholecystokinin; FAs, fatty acids; H+, hydrogen ion; HCO_3^-, bicarbonate; H_2O, water.

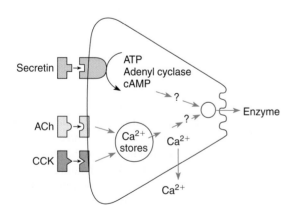

FIGURE 9-8 ■ Receptors on the rodent pancreatic acinar cell. Different second messengers for the stimulants indicate different cellular mechanisms for stimulation and provide the basis for potentiation. ACh, acetylcholine; ATP, adenosine triphosphate; Ca^{2+}, calcium; cAMP, cyclic adenosine monophosphate; CCK, cholecystokinin.

RESPONSE TO A MEAL

As digestion and mixing of food proceed in the stomach, buffers present in proteins and peptides become saturated with H+, and the pH drops to approximately 2. The maximum load of titratable acid (free H+ plus bound H+) delivered to the duodenum is 20 to 30 mEq/hour. This is approximately equal to the maximal capacity of the stomach to secrete acid, which, in turn, equals the ability of the pancreas to secrete HCO_3^- when it is maximally stimulated. To raise the pH of the duodenum, the undissociated H+, as well as the free H+, must be neutralized. This is accomplished rapidly in the first part of the duodenum, and the pH of the chyme is raised quickly from 2 at the pylorus to more than 4 beyond the duodenal bulb. Some neutralization occurs by absorption of H+ and secretion of HCO_3^- by the gut wall. An additional amount of H+ is neutralized by HCO_3^- in the bile. The contributions of the gut mucosa and bile are small, however, and the greatest proportion of acid by far is neutralized by the large volume of pancreatic juice secreted into the lumen.

Within a few minutes after chyme enters the duodenum, a sharp rise in the secretion of pancreatic enzymes occurs. Within 30 minutes, enzyme secretion peaks at levels approximately 70% to 80% of those attainable with maximal stimulation by CCK and cholinergic reflexes. Enzyme secretion continues at this rate until the stomach is empty. The enzyme response to a meal may be kept below maximum by the presence of humoral inhibitors of pancreatic secretion. This is the proposed function of pancreatic polypeptide.

Pancreatic enzyme secretion is able to adapt to the diet. In other words, ingestion of a high-protein, low-carbohydrate diet over several days increases the proportion of proteases and decreases the proportion of amylase in pancreatic juice. This type of response is now known to be hormonally regulated at the level of gene expression. CCK increases the expression of the genes for proteases and decreases the expression for amylase. Secretin and gastric inhibitory peptide (GIP) increase the expression of the gene for lipase. The mechanism to increase amylase gene expression under normal conditions is not known, although insulin regulates amylase levels in diabetes.

Insulin potentiates the secretory responses to CCK and secretin, a finding that probably accounts for the reduced pancreatic enzyme secretion in human diabetic patients who have no obvious pancreatic disease. Insulin also is necessary to maintain normal rates of pancreatic protein synthesis and stores of digestive enzymes.

CLINICAL APPLICATIONS

Abnormal pancreatic secretion occurs with diseases such as chronic and acute pancreatitis, cystic fibrosis, and kwashiorkor, as well as with tumors that involve the gland itself. Changes in secretion during the course of one of these diseases depend on the stage of development of the disease. Most patients with **chronic pancreatitis** have decreased volume and bicarbonate output, whereas those with acute pancreatitis often have normal secretion. Both volume and enzyme content of pancreatic juice are decreased by cystic fibrosis. **Tumors of the pancreas** frequently decrease the volume of secretion. In **kwashiorkor**, severe protein deficiency, the alkaline and enzymatic components are depressed, but amylase secretion continues after trypsin, chymotrypsin, and lipase activities are no longer found.

Pancreatitis is an inflammatory disease of the pancreas that occurs when proteases are activated within the acinar cells. These enzymes are synthesized in inactive forms and normally are activated only when they reach the intestine. The most common causes of this condition are excessive alcohol consumption and blockage of the pancreatic duct. Blockage is usually the result of gallstones and frequently occurs at the ampulla of Vater. Secretions build up behind the obstruction, and trypsin accumulates and activates other pancreatic proteases, as well as additional trypsin. Eventually, the normal defense mechanisms are overwhelmed, and pancreatic tissue is digested. In addition to synthesizing proteases as inactive proenzymes, the pancreas has several other mechanisms to prevent damage. First, enzymes are membrane bound from the time of synthesis until they are secreted from zymogen granules. Second, acinar cells contain a trypsin inhibitor, which destroys activated enzymes. Third, trypsin itself is capable of autodigestion. Fourth, some lysosomal enzymes also degrade activated zymogens. Approximately 10% of pancreatitis cases are hereditary. Mutations associated with the normal defense mechanisms have been identified as accounting for most of these cases. Two mutations occur in the trypsin gene itself. One (R122H) enhances trypsin activity by impairing its autodigestion. The other (N29I) leads to an increased rate of autoactivation. In addition, mutations in the native trypsin inhibitor have been shown to increase the risk of disease.

Cystic fibrosis is characterized by decreased chloride (Cl^-) secretion of many epithelial tissues and the inability of cyclic adenosine monophosphate (cAMP) to regulate Cl^- conductance. As mentioned earlier, good evidence indicates that

Continued

CLINICAL APPLICATIONS—cont'd

the ion channel for Cl^- in the apical membrane of the duct cell is the cystic fibrosis transmembrane conductance regulator that is regulated by cAMP. Failure to synthesize this protein in its normal state or failure to insert it properly in the apical membrane results in cystic fibrosis and a severe decrease of ductal secretion. As a result, proteinaceous acinar secretions become concentrated and precipitate within the duct lumen, thus blocking small ducts and eventually destroying the gland.

Pancreatic enzyme secretion must be reduced by more than 80% to produce **steatorrhea.** If a patient has steatorrhea, it is necessary only to measure the concentration of any pancreatic enzyme in the jejunal content after a meal to determine whether the condition is pancreatic in origin.

Pancreatic exocrine function is assessed by measuring basal secretion and secretion stimulated by secretin and/or cholecystokinin (CCK). These function tests are performed on a fasting patient. A double-lumen nasogastric tube is used. One tube opens into the stomach to drain gastric contents that would otherwise empty into the duodenum; the other collects duodenal juice that is assumed to be largely pancreatic in origin. Interpretation of the test is impeded by contaminating biliary secretions. Changes in secretion depend on the stage of development of various diseases and may vary from patient to patient. For these reasons, pancreatic function tests are not reliable in the diagnosis of individual diseases but are used to assess overall pancreatic function.

SUMMARY

1. Pancreatic secretion consists of an aqueous HCO_3^- component from the duct cells and an enzymatic component from the acinar cells.
2. The duct cells actively secrete HCO_3^- into the lumen, and Na^+ and water follow down electrical and osmotic gradients, respectively.
3. The composition of pancreatic juice varies with the rate of secretion. At low rates, Na^+ and Cl^- predominate; at high rates, Na^+ and HCO_3^- predominate.
4. Pancreatic enzymes are essential for the digestion of all major foodstuffs and are stored in zymogen granules of acinar cells before secretion.
5. The primary stimulant of the aqueous component is secretin, whose effects are potentiated by CCK and ACh.
6. During the cephalic phase of secretion, vagal stimulation results in a low volume of secretion containing a high concentration of enzymes. This secretion is produced by the acinar cells.
7. During the intestinal phase, acid (pH less than 4.5) releases secretin. Fats and amino acids release CCK, which activates vagal afferents. The resulting vagovagal reflexes mediated by ACh stimulate enzyme secretion from the acinar cells. Stimulants using different second messengers potentiate each other.

KEY WORDS AND CONCEPTS

Aqueous component

Enzymatic/protein component

Acinar cells

Ductule cells

Centroacinar cells

Islets of Langerhans

Potentiation

Chronic pancreatitis

Tumors of the pancreas

Kwashiorkor

Cystic fibrosis

Steatorrhea

SUGGESTED READINGS

Anagostides A, Chadwick VS, Selden AC, et al: Sham feeding and pancreatic secretion: evidence for direct vagal stimulation of enzyme output, *Gastroenterology* 87:109–114, 1984.

Argent BE, Gray MA, Steward MC, Case RM: Cell physiology of pancreatic ducts. In Johnson LR, editor: ed 5, *Physiology of the Gastrointestinal Tract*, vol 2, San Diego, 2012, Elsevier.

Gorelick FS, Jamieson JD: Structure-function relationships in the pancreatic acinar cell. In Johnson LR, editor: ed 5, *Physiology of the Gastrointestinal Tract*, vol 2, San Diego, 2012, Elsevier.

Jensen RT: Receptors on pancreatic acinar cells. In Johnson LR, editor: ed 3, *Physiology of the Gastrointestinal Tract*, New York, 1994, Raven Press.

Ji B, Bi Y, Simeone D, et al: Human pancreatic acinar cells lack functional responses to cholecystokinin and gastrin, *Gastroenterology* 121:1380–1390, 2001.

Logsdon CD: Pancreatic enzyme secretion (physiology). In Johnson LR, editor: *Encyclopedia of Gastroenterology*, vol 3, San Diego, 2004, Academic Press, pp 68–75.

Meyer JH, Way LW, Grossman MI: Pancreatic response to acidification of various lengths of proximal intestine in the dog, *Am J Physiol* 219:971–977, 1970.

Liddle RA: Regulation of pancreatic secretion. In Johnson LR, editor: ed 5, *Physiology of the Gastrointestinal Tract*, vol 2, San Diego, 2012, Elsevier.

Solomon TE, Grossman MI: Effect of atropine and vagotomy on response of transplanted pancreas, *Am J Physiol* 236:E186–E190, 1979.

Williams JA, Yule DI: Stimulus-secretion coupling in the pancreatic acinar cells. In Johnson LR, editor: ed 5, *Physiology of the Gastrointestinal Tract*, vol 2, San Diego, 2012, Elsevier.

10

BILE SECRETION AND GALLBLADDER FUNCTION

■ ■ ■ ■ ■ ■ ■

OBJECTIVES

- Describe the constituents of bile and their functions.
- Understand the solubility of the bile acids and bile salts and how it affects their reabsorption in the small bowel.
- Describe the enterohepatic circulation and its role in bile acid synthesis and the secretion of bile.
- Understand the process involved in the excretion of bile pigments and its relationship with jaundice.
- Explain the function of the gallbladder.
- Describe the regulation of bile secretion from the liver and its expulsion from the gallbladder.
- Explain the abnormalities that may lead to the formation of gallstones.

B ile is responsible for the principal digestive functions of the liver. Bile in the small intestine is necessary for the digestion and absorption of lipids. The problem of the insolubility of fats in water is solved by the constituents of bile. The bile salts and other organic components of bile are responsible in part for emulsifying fat so that it can be digested by pancreatic lipase. The bile acids also take part in solubilizing the digestion products into micelles. Micellar formation is essential for the optimal absorption of fat digestion products. Bile also serves as the vehicle for the elimination of a variety of substances from the body. These include endogenous products such as cholesterol and bile pigments, as well as some drugs and heavy metals.

OVERVIEW OF THE BILIARY SYSTEM

Figure 10-1 is a schematic illustration of the biliary system and the circulation of bile acids between the intestine and liver. **Bile** is continuously produced by the hepatocytes. The principal organic constituents of bile are the **bile acids,** which are synthesized by the hepatocytes. The secretion of bile acids carries water and electrolytes into the bile by osmotic filtration. Additional water and electrolytes, primarily sodium bicarbonate ($NaHCO_3$), are added by cells lining the ducts. This latter component is stimulated by secretin and is essentially identical to the aqueous component of pancreatic secretion. The secretion of bile increases pressure in the hepatic ducts and causes the gallbladder to fill. Within the gallbladder, bile is stored and concentrated by the absorption of water and electrolytes. When a meal is eaten, the gallbladder is stimulated to contract by CCK and vagal stimulation. Within the lumen of the intestine bile participates in the emulsification, hydrolysis, and absorption of lipids. Most bile acids are absorbed either passively throughout the intestine or actively in the ileum. Bile acids lost in the feces are replaced by synthesis in the hepatocytes. The absorbed bile acids are returned to the liver via the portal circulation, where they are extracted actively from the blood. Together with newly synthesized bile acids, the returning bile acids are secreted into the bile canaliculi. Canalicular bile is secreted by ductule cells in response to the osmotic effects of anion transport. In humans, almost all bile

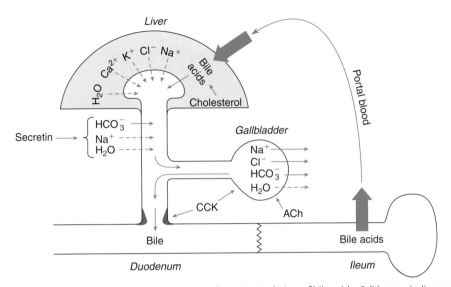

FIGURE 10-1 ■ Overview of the biliary system and the enterohepatic circulation of bile acids. *Solid arrows* indicate active transport processes. ACh, acetylcholine; Ca^{2+}, calcium; CCK, cholecystokinin; Cl^-, chloride; H^+, hydrogen ion; HCO_3^-, bicarbonate; H_2O, water; K^+, potassium; Na^+, sodium. *(From Johnson LR: Essential Medical Physiology, 3rd ed. Philadelphia, Academic Press, 2003, p 521.)*

formation is driven by bile acids and is therefore referred to as **bile acid dependent.** The portion of bile stimulated by secretin and contributed by the ducts is termed **bile acid independent** or **ductular secretion.**

CONSTITUENTS OF BILE

Bile is a complex mixture of organic and inorganic components. Taken separately, some of the components are insoluble and would precipitate out of an aqueous medium. Normally, however, bile is a homogeneous and stable solution whose stability depends on the physical behavior and interactions of its various components.

Bile acids, the major organic constituents of bile, account for approximately 50% of the solid components. Chemically, they are carboxylic acids with a cyclopentanoperhydrophenanthrene nucleus and a branched side chain of three to nine carbon atoms that ends in a carboxyl group (Fig. 10-2). They are related structurally to cholesterol, from which they are synthesized by the liver. Indeed, the synthesis of bile acids is a major pathway for the elimination of cholesterol from the body. Conversion of cholesterol to bile acids occurs via two main synthetic pathways.

The major pathway begins with the rate-limiting step of 7α-hydroxylation of cholesterol by the hepatic enzyme

7α-hydroxylase. A secondary pathway begins with the conversion of cholesterol to 27-hydroxycholesterol, a reaction that takes place in many tissues. Four bile acids are present in bile, along with trace amounts of others that are modifications of the four. The liver synthesizes two bile acids, **cholic acid** and **chenodeoxycholic acid.** These are the primary bile acids (see Fig. 10-2). Within the lumen of the gut, a fraction of each acid is dehydroxylated by bacteria to form **deoxycholic acid** and **lithocholic acid.** These are called secondary bile acids. All four are returned to the liver in the portal blood and are secreted into the bile. Their relative amounts in bile are approximately four cholic to two chenodeoxycholic acid to one deoxycholic to only small amounts of lithocholic acid.

The solubility of bile acids depends on the number of hydroxyl groups present and the state of the terminal carboxyl group. Cholic acid, with three hydroxyl groups, is the most soluble, whereas lithocholic, a monohydroxy acid, is least soluble. The dissociation constant (pK) of the bile acids is near the pH of the duodenal contents, so there are relatively equal amounts of protonated (insoluble) forms and ionic (soluble) forms. The liver, however, conjugates the bile acids to the amino acids glycine or taurine with a pKa of 3.7 and 1.5, respectively. Thus at the pH of

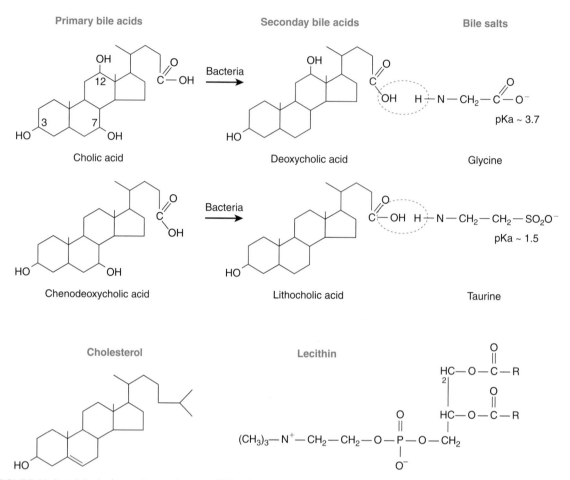

FIGURE 10-2 ■ Principal organic constituents of bile. The two primary bile acids may be converted to secondary bile acids in the intestine. Each of the four bile acids may be conjugated to either glycine or taurine to form bile salts. The R-groups of lecithin represent fatty acids. pKa, negative log of dissociation constant. *(From Johnson LR: Essential Medical Physiology, 3rd ed. Philadelphia, Academic Press, 2003, p 522.)*

duodenal contents, bile acids are largely ionized and water soluble. Conjugated bile acids exist as salts of various cations, primarily Na$^+$, and are referred to as **bile salts** (see Fig. 10-2).

Several features are unique to the bile acids and account for their behavior in solution. Three-dimensionally, the hydroxyl and carboxyl groups are located on one side of the molecule. The bulk of the molecule is composed of the nucleus and several methyl groups (Fig. 10-3). This structure renders bile acids amphipathic to the extent that the hydroxyl groups, the peptide bond of the side chain, and either the carbonyl or

sulfonyl group of glycine or taurine are hydrophilic, and the cholesterol nucleus and methyl groupings are hydrophobic. In solution, the behavior of bile acids depends on their concentration. At low concentrations, little interaction occurs among bile acid molecules. As the concentration is increased, a point is reached at which aggregation of the molecules takes place. These aggregates are called **micelles,** and the point of formation is called the **critical micellar concentration.** Hydrophobic regions of the micelles interact with one another, and the hydrophilic regions interact with the water molecules (see Fig. 10-3).

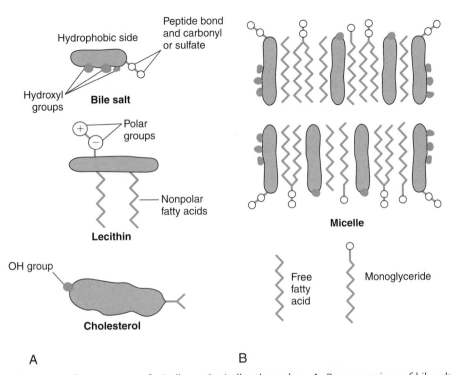

FIGURE 10-3 ■ Structures of components of micelles and micelles themselves. **A,** Representations of bile salt, lecithin, and cholesterol molecules illustrating the separation of polar and nonpolar surfaces. **B,** Cross section of a micelle showing the arrangement of these molecules and the principal products of fat digestion. Micelles are cylindrical disks whose outer curved surfaces are composed of bile salts. OH, hydroxyl. *(From Johnson LR: Essential Medical Physiology, 3rd ed. Philadelphia, Academic Press, 2003, p 523.)*

The second most abundant group of organic compounds in bile consists of the **phospholipids,** and the major ones are the lecithins (see Fig. 10-3). Phospholipids also are amphipathic, insofar as the phosphatidylcholine grouping is hydrophilic, whereas the fatty acid chains are hydrophobic. Although amphipathic, the phospholipids are not soluble in water but form liquid crystals that swell in solution. In the presence of bile salts, however, the liquid crystals are broken up and solubilized as a component of the micelles. Bile salts possess a large capacity to solubilize phospholipids; 2 moles (mol) of lecithin are solubilized by 1 mol of bile salts. The combination of bile salts and phospholipids also is better able to solubilize other lipids—mainly cholesterol and the products of fat digestion—than is a simple solution of bile salts.

A third organic component, **cholesterol,** is present in small amounts and contributes approximately 4% to the total solids of bile. Although present in small amounts, bile cholesterol is important because it may be excreted and therefore helps regulate body stores of cholesterol. Cholesterol appears mainly in the nonesterified form and is insoluble in water. In the presence of bile salts and phospholipids, however, it is solubilized as part of the micelle. Because it is a weakly polar substance, cholesterol is found in the interior of the micelle, where the hydrophobic portions of the bile salts, phospholipids, monoglycerides, and fatty acids interact (see Fig. 10-3). Within the liver, ducts, and gallbladder, bile is normally present as a micellar solution.

The fourth major group of organic compounds found in bile comprises the **bile pigments.** These constitute only 2% of the total solids, and bilirubin is the most important. Chemically, bile pigments are tetrapyrroles and are related to the porphyrins, from which they are derived. In their free form, bile pigments are insoluble in water. Normally, however, they are conjugated with glucuronic acid and are rendered soluble. Unlike the other organic compounds just mentioned, bile pigments do not take part in micellar formation. As their name implies, they are highly colored substances. Other than being responsible for the normal color of bile and feces, the pigment properties of these compounds are used to assess the level of function of the liver.

In addition to the organic compounds just discussed, many **inorganic ions** are found in bile. The predominant cation is Na^+, accompanied by smaller amounts of potassium (K^+) and calcium (Ca^{2+}). The predominant inorganic anions are chloride (Cl^-) and HCO_3^-. Normally, the total number of inorganic cations exceeds the total number of inorganic anions. No anion deficit occurs, however, because the bile acids, which possess a net negative charge at the pH values found in bile, account for the difference. Bile is isosmotic even though the number of cations present is larger than expected. Because they are highly charged molecules, the bile acids attract a layer of cations that serve as counterions. These counterions are tightly associated with the micelles and thus exert little osmotic activity.

BILE SECRETION

Functional Histology of the Liver

The functional organization of the liver is shown schematically in Figure 10-4. The liver is divided into lobules organized around a central vein that receives blood through separations surrounded by plates of hepatocytes. The separations are called sinusoids, and they in turn are supplied by blood from both the portal vein and the hepatic artery. The plates of hepatocytes are no more than two cells thick, so every hepatocyte is exposed to blood. Openings between the plates ensure that the blood is exposed to a large surface area. The hepatocytes remove substances from the blood and secrete them into the biliary canaliculi lying between the adjacent hepatocytes. The bile flows toward the periphery, countercurrent to the flow of the blood, and drains into bile ducts. This countercurrent relationship minimizes the concentration differences between substances in the blood and in the bile and contributes to the liver's efficiency in extracting substances from the blood.

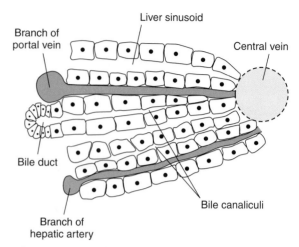

FIGURE 10-4 ■ Schematic diagram of the relationship between blood vessels, hepatocytes, and bile canaliculi in the liver. Each hepatocyte is exposed to blood at one membrane surface and a bile canaliculus at the other. *(From Johnson LR: Essential Medical Physiology, 3rd ed. Philadelphia, Academic Press, 2003, p 524.)*

Bile Acids and the Enterohepatic Circulation

The secretion of bile depends heavily on the secretion of bile acids by the liver. Once secreted, bile acids undergo an interesting journey (see Fig. 10-1). First, they may be stored in the gallbladder. Then they are propelled into and through the small intestine, where they take part in the digestion and absorption of lipids. Most of the bile acids themselves are absorbed from the intestine and travel via the portal blood to the liver, where they are taken up by the hepatocytes and resecreted. This process is termed the **enterohepatic circulation.**

Bile acids are secreted continuously by the liver. The rate of secretion, however, varies widely. Early experiments demonstrated that the rate of secretion depended on the amount of bile acids delivered to the liver via the blood; the more acids in the portal blood, the greater the secretion of bile. The amount of bile acids in the portal blood depends on the amount absorbed from the small intestine. The amount of bile acids in the intestine, in turn, depends on the digestive state of the individual. Between meals, most bile secreted by the liver is stored in the gallbladder, with only small amounts delivered intermittently to the small intestine. During a meal, the gallbladder empties

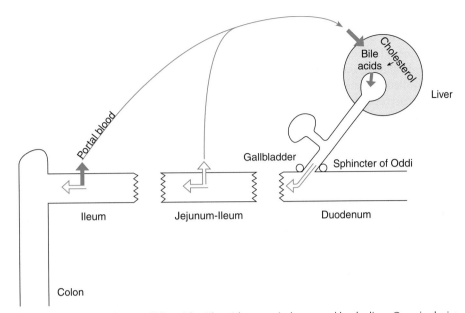

FIGURE 10-5 ■ Enterohepatic circulation of bile acids. Bile acids are actively secreted by the liver. Once in the intestine they participate in the digestion and absorption of lipids. As they are propelled toward the distal small bowel, some of the "primary" acids are altered and become "secondary" acids. The more hydrophobic bile acids are absorbed passively throughout the intestine. The more hydrophilic acids are absorbed by a sodium-coupled active transport process that is localized to the ileum. A minor fraction of bile acids is not absorbed but is instead propelled into the colon. The absorbed bile acids are transported via the portal circulation to the liver, where they are extracted actively from the blood (at a rate of almost 100%) and resecreted. Synthesis of new primary acids from cholesterol occurs at a rate to compensate for the acids lost from the bowel. *Solid arrows* denote active absorption, secretion, and synthesis; *open arrows* denote passive absorption and propulsion of contents by contractions of the intestine.

its contents into the duodenum in a more continuous pattern. The ejected bile acids are then resorbed from the intestine and are secreted again by the liver.

Although many different bile acids are found in the bile, only cholic acid and chenodeoxycholic acid appear to be synthesized from cholesterol in significant amounts by human hepatocytes. For this reason, they are called "primary" bile acids. Their synthesis by the liver is a continuous but regulated process. The amount synthesized depends on the amount of bile acids returned to the liver in the enterohepatic circulation. When most of the bile acids secreted by the liver are returned, synthesis is low, but when the secreted acids are lost from the enterohepatic circulation, the rate of synthesis is high. Bile acids extracted from the portal blood act to feedback inhibit 7α-hydroxylase, the rate-limiting enzyme for the synthesis of bile acids from cholesterol. Normally, there are 2.5 g of bile salts in the enterohepatic circulation. If the absorptive processes in the intestine and liver are functioning properly, only

approximately 0.5 g is lost daily. Synthesis is regulated to replenish this loss. If the enterohepatic circulation is interrupted (e.g., by a fistula draining bile to the outside), the rate of synthesis becomes maximal. In humans, this amounts to 3 to 5 g per day. In patients incapable of reabsorbing bile acids, the maximal rate of synthesis equals the total amount of bile acids secreted by the liver. Deoxycholic acid, lithocholic acid, and other "secondary" bile acids are produced in the intestine through the action of microorganisms on primary bile acids. These acids then are absorbed along with the primary bile acids, taken up by the hepatocytes, conjugated with taurine and glycine, and secreted in the bile. The bile acid pool may circulate through the enterohepatic circulation several times during the digestion of a meal, so that 15 to 30 g bile acids may enter the duodenum during a 24-hour period.

The enterohepatic circulation of bile acids is carried out by both active and passive transport processes (Fig. 10-5). The more hydrophobic bile acids, which are those with fewer hydroxyl groups and those that have been deconjugated, are absorbed passively throughout the intestine. The more hydrophilic acids and the remaining hydrophobic acids are absorbed by an active process in the ileum. Uptake across the apical membrane of the enterocytes is mediated by a specific Na^+-dependent transport protein. Cytoplasmic binding proteins transport the acids through the cell to the basolateral membrane. Transport across the basolateral membrane out of the cell is mediated by an Na^+-independent anion exchange process that involves a carrier different from the one on the apical membrane. As stated previously, the ileal transport process is highly efficient, delivering more than 90% of the bile acids to the portal blood.

In the liver, additional transport processes remove bile acids from the portal blood. Uptake across the basolateral or sinusoidal membrane of the enterocytes is mediated primarily by two types of systems. One group includes a specific Na^+-coupled transporter protein, the Na^+ taurocholate cotransporting polypeptide (**NTCP**), which can transfer both conjugated and unconjugated bile acids. A group of Na^+-independent transporters includes the organic anion transport proteins (**OATPs**), which can take up both bile acids and other organic anions. At the canaliculus, bile acids and other organic anions appear to be secreted by at least two adenosine triphosphate (ATP)-dependent processes. One of these is termed the *bile salt excretory pump* (**bsep**), and the other is the *multidrug resistance protein 2* (**mrp2**). The hepatic transport of bile acids also is highly efficient. Practically all bile acids contained in the portal blood are removed during one passage through the liver. The process does have a transport maximum, but this is seldom reached.

Cholesterol and Phospholipids

Cholesterol and phospholipids, primarily lecithins, also are secreted by the hepatocytes. The exact mechanisms of secretion are not known, but secretion appears to depend, in part, on the secretion of bile acids. The higher the rate of bile acid secretion is, the higher the rate of cholesterol and phospholipid secretion will be. Once secreted into the intestine along with the other components of bile, cholesterol and lecithin are mixed with and handled as ingested cholesterol and lecithin (see Chapter 11).

Bilirubin

The primary bile pigment in humans, **bilirubin,** is derived largely from the metabolic breakdown of **hemoglobin** (Fig. 10-6). Most of the hemoglobin comes from aged red blood cells (RBCs) that are disposed of by cells of the reticuloendothelial (RE) system. In the RE cells, hemoglobin is split into hemin and globin. The hemin ring is opened and oxidized, and the iron is removed to form bilirubin, which is then transported via the blood from the cells of the RE system to the hepatocytes. In transit, bilirubin is tightly bound to plasma albumin; very little is free in the plasma. Hepatocytes can extract bilirubin from blood, conjugate it with glucuronic acid, and secrete the conjugated product into the bile. Bilirubin secretion into the bile by the hepatocytes is mediated by an active anion transport system. This system is different from the one for active transport of bile acids, but it is shared by certain other organic anions (e.g., sulfobromophthalein [Bromsulphalein, or BSP], various radiopaque dyes). Some evidence indicates that one of the OATPs participates in the transport of bilirubin.

Bilirubin is not absorbed from the intestine in any appreciable amount. Some of the product, however, is altered in the bowel. Bacteria, primarily in the distal small bowel and colon, reduce bilirubin to urobilinogen, which is unconjugated. Some urobilinogen is converted to stercobilin and is excreted in the feces. Urobilinogen also is absorbed into the portal blood and returned to the liver. There most is extracted, conjugated, and secreted into the bile; however, some passes into the systemic circulation and is excreted by the kidneys. The urobilinogen is oxidized in the urine to form urobilin. Stercobilin and urobilin are pigments that are in large part responsible for the color of the feces and urine, respectively. Following damage to the liver, sufficient bilirubin may not be extracted, and the skin takes on a yellow tinge. This condition, termed **jaundice,** is usually especially noticeable in the eyes. Bilirubin is also responsible for the yellow color that bruises develop after several days.

Water and Electrolytes

Two components of bile water and electrolyte secretion have been identified. One is called **bile acid–dependent secretion.** Bile acids, regardless of

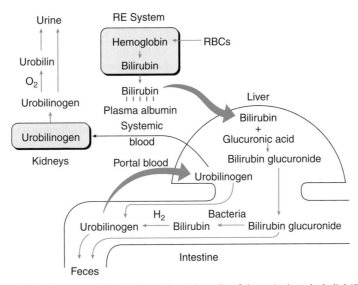

FIGURE 10-6 ■ Excretion of bile pigments. Bilirubin is produced by cells of the reticuloendothelial (RE) system from aged red blood cells (RBCs). The unconjugated pigment is then carried, tightly bound to plasma albumin, to the liver. There it is actively taken up, conjugated with glucuronic acid, and secreted into the bile. The water-soluble conjugates are propelled along the intestine. In the distal small bowel and colon a portion of the conjugated pigment is acted on by bacteria and becomes unconjugated bilirubin and other pigments. Some of these pigments are absorbed passively into the blood and either returned to the liver and resecreted or passed through the liver and excreted by the kidneys. Most, however, pass through the colon and are excreted. *Bold arrows* indicate active absorption. H_2, hydrogen.

whether they are newly synthesized or extracted from the portal blood, are the major component actively secreted by the hepatocytes. Because they are anions, their secretion is accompanied by the passive movement of cations into the canaliculus, which in turn sets up an osmotic gradient down which water moves (Fig. 10-7). Canalicular bile is thus primarily an ultrafiltrate of plasma as far as the concentrations of water are concerned. In some species, although not proven in humans, there is evidence for the active transport of Na^+ by the hepatocytes. The higher the rate of return of bile acids is to the liver, the faster they are secreted and the greater is the volume of bile.

The contribution of the bile ducts and ductules to bile production is identical to that of the pancreatic ducts to pancreatic juice. Secretin stimulates the secretion of HCO_3^- and water from the ductile cells, thereby resulting in a significant increase in bile volume, HCO_3^- concentration, and pH and a decrease in the concentration of bile salts. The mechanism of HCO_3^- secretion by the ducts of the liver involves active transport and is similar to the mechanism employed by the pancreas.

When stimulated by secretin, the HCO_3^- concentration of the bile may increase two- or threefold over that of plasma. This fraction of secretion is called the **bile acid–independent** or the **secretin-dependent** portion.

GALLBLADDER FUNCTION

Filling

The primary force responsible for the flow of bile from the canaliculi toward the small intestine is the secretory pressure generated by the hepatocytes and ductule epithelium. The hepatic end of the biliary tract is blind, formed by the secretory cells of the liver. Thus as bile is secreted by these cells, pressure in the ducts rises. The active secretion of bile acids and electrolytes can make biliary secretory pressures reach a level of 10 to 20 millimeters of mercury (mm Hg).

Whether bile flows into the duodenum or into the gallbladder depends on a balance between resistance to the filling of the gallbladder and resistance to bile flowing through the terminal **bile duct** and **sphincter of Oddi.** The gallbladder is a distensible muscular organ that forms a blind outpouching of the biliary

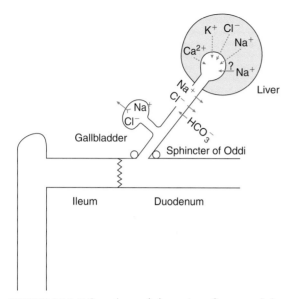

FIGURE 10-7 ■ Secretion and absorption of water and electrolytes. The osmotic gradient created by the active secretion of bile acids, and perhaps sodium (Na^+), causes water to move from the hepatocytes into the bile canaliculi. Ions accompany water movement, presumably via the process of bulk flow. Epithelial cells of the bile ducts are capable of actively absorbing Na^+ and chloride (Cl^-) and of actively secreting Na^+ and bicarbonate (HCO_3^-). In the gallbladder, salt absorption is accompanied by the absorption of water, thus concentrating the bile.

tract. Its inner surface is lined with a thin layer of epithelial cells having high absorptive capacity. The sphincter of Oddi is a thickening of the circular muscle of the bile duct located at the ductal entrance into the duodenum. Although this muscle is embedded in the wall of the duodenum, it appears to be an entity separate from the duodenal musculature. Most of the time during fasting, the gallbladder is readily distensible, and the sphincter of Oddi maintains closure of the terminal bile duct. Thus bile secreted by the liver flows into the gallbladder (Fig. 10-8).

Concentration of the Bile

The human gallbladder is not a large organ and, when full, can accommodate only 20 to 50 mL of fluid. During fasting, however, many times that volume of fluid may be secreted by the liver. The discrepancy between the amount of bile secreted by the liver and the amount stored in the gallbladder is accounted for by the

gallbladder's ability to concentrate bile. The concentration of bile salts, bile pigments, and other large water-soluble molecules may increase by a factor of 5 to 20 as a result of water and electrolyte absorption.

Absorption of water and electrolytes is partly an active process. Na^+ absorption can occur against an electrochemical gradient, is a saturable process, depends on metabolic activity, and demonstrates other characteristics of an active transport mechanism. Unlike the transport mechanisms for Na^+ that exist in other epithelia, however, transport in the gallbladder is not associated with the generation of any measurable electrical potential difference. In addition, it is highly dependent on the presence of either Cl^- or HCO_3^-. Thus it appears as though Na^+ transport is coupled with the transport of an anion and is electrically neutral.

As in other epithelial tissues, water movement in the gallbladder depends on the active absorption of NaCl and $NaHCO_3$ and thus is entirely passive. The rows of epithelial cells of the mucosa have large lateral intercellular spaces near the basal membrane and possess tight junctions at cell apices. Solute is transported actively from the cells into the intercellular space at the apical ends. This movement is then followed by the passive diffusion of water. The movement of water molecules, however, is such that an osmotic gradient is set up in the intercellular spaces. The solution is hypertonic at the apical end and isotonic at the basal end. In the steady state, this standing osmotic gradient is maintained and accounts for the absorption of a solution with fixed osmolality.

Absorption of Na^+, Cl^-, HCO_3^-, and water influences the concentrations of other solutes in the bile. Ions such as K^+ and Ca^{2+} become more concentrated. The concentration of bile salts also increases during the absorption of water and electrolytes, often to the point of the critical micellar concentration. The presence of micelles, which have minimal osmotic activity, permits the high concentration of electrolytes, bile salts, phospholipids, and cholesterol to be isotonic in gallbladder bile (Table 10-1).

EXPULSION OF BILE

Most bile secretion occurs during the digestion of meals. However, significant amounts are secreted

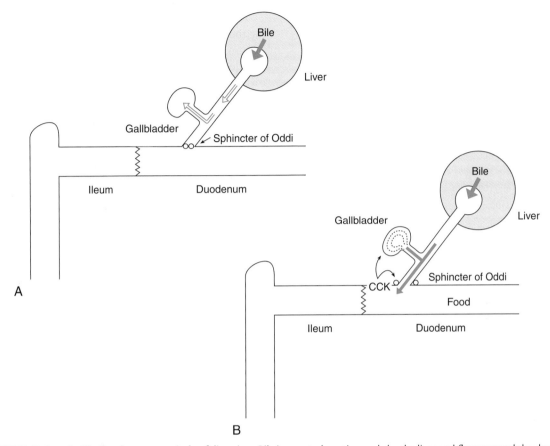

FIGURE 10-8 ■ A, Bile flow between periods of digestion. Bile is secreted continuously by the liver and flows toward the duodenum. In the interdigestive period the gallbladder is readily distensible, and the sphincter of Oddi is contracted. Therefore, bile flows into the gallbladder rather than the duodenum. **B,** On eating, both hormonal (e.g., cholecystokinin [CCK]) and neural stimuli cause contraction of the gallbladder and relaxation of the sphincter of Oddi. Thus, bile flows into the bowel. Bile secretion from the liver increases as bile acids are returned via the enterohepatic circulation.

periodically during fasting in synchrony with the migrating motor complex (MMC). The gallbladder contracts, expelling bile, shortly before and during the period of intense sequential duodenal contractions. Thus bile, along with other secretions, is swept aborally along the bowel by these contractions. The exact stimuli and pathways responsible for coordinating gallbladder contraction with cyclic intestinal motility are not known, but they appear to involve cholinergic nerves.

Shortly after eating, the gallbladder musculature contracts rhythmically and empties gradually (see Fig. 10-8, *B*). The stimulus for its contraction appears to be primarily hormonal. Products of food digestion, particularly lipids, release **cholecystokinin** (CCK) from the mucosa of the duodenum. This hormone is carried in the blood to the gallbladder, where it stimulates the musculature to contract. CCK is a stimulant of gallbladder muscle and may act in part by binding to receptors located directly on smooth muscle cells. In vivo, however, much of the action of CCK appears to be mediated through extrinsic vagal and intrinsic cholinergic nerves. The role of other gastrointestinal hormones is less clear. Gastrin stimulates gallbladder contraction, but in doses that are well above the physiologic range. Secretin appears to have little direct effect on the gallbladder, although it may antagonize (or prevent) the effects of CCK. Pancreatic polypeptide and somatostatin both have been shown to decrease

TABLE 10-1

Approximate Values for Major Components of Liver and Gallbladder Bile

Component	Liver Bile	Gallbladder Bile
Na^+ (mmol/L)	150	300
K^+ (mmol/L)	4.5	10
Ca^{2+} (mmol/L)	4	20
Cl^- (mmol/L)	80	5
Bile salts (mmol/L)	30	315
pH	7.4	6.5
Cholesterol (mg/100 mL)	110	600
Bilirubin (mg/100 mL)	100	1000

Reprinted with permission from Johnson LR: Essential Medical Physiology, 3rd ed. Philadelphia, Academic Press, 2003.

gallbladder contractility and may affect gallbladder function in certain disease states.

The flow of bile from the gallbladder through the common bile duct and into the duodenum is influenced by muscular activity of the common bile duct, sphincter of Oddi, and duodenum. The bile duct contains smooth muscle cells, and measurements of its contractile activity have been made in certain species. Some investigators maintain that peristaltic contractions of the duct do occur, and that these facilitate movement of bile into the duodenum. The relative importance of this mechanism is not known.

The sphincter of Oddi is a muscular ring surrounding the opening of the bile duct in the wall of the duodenum. Its relative contributions to the regulation of bile flow sometimes are difficult to assess because its own activity is influenced by the musculature of the duodenum. The sphincter can maintain closure of the bile duct independently of activity of the duodenal musculature. When the duodenum is relaxed, pressures of 12 to 30 mm Hg are needed to force fluid through a closed sphincter. However, bile flow through an open sphincter of Oddi is influenced markedly by the contractile activity of the duodenum. Bile enters an actively contracting bowel in spurts during periods of duodenal relaxation and stops during periods of contraction. The sphincter, like the muscle of the gallbladder, is controlled by the hormone CCK. In contrast to its action on the gallbladder, CCK relaxes the sphincter of Oddi and thereby allows bile to enter the duodenum. In a manner similar to its mechanism of action on the gallbladder, CCK appears to influence sphincter of Oddi function by acting on nerves, rather than directly on smooth muscle.

The role of the autonomic nervous system in the control of bile flow is not clear. Stimulation of parasympathetic nerves causes an increase in bile flow and contraction of the gallbladder. Stimulation of sympathetic nerves has the opposite effect. Bile flow begins shortly after eating and may be part of the cephalic phase of digestion. The emotional state of the person also has been shown to influence bile flow.

CLINICAL APPLICATIONS

Abnormalities of bile secretion can result from functional changes in the liver, bile ducts, gallbladder, and intestine. Because many of the components of bile are synthesized and/or actively secreted by hepatocytes, metabolic abnormalities of these cells can result in decreased bile production and increased plasma levels of those constituents normally excreted in the bile (e.g., bile acids, bile pigments). Metabolic abnormalities more commonly result from the destruction of hepatocytes by infectious agents (e.g., viral hepatitis) and various toxins. However, several conditions are characterized by genetic deficiencies in one or more of the steps of bilirubin secretion. These deficiencies also can result in **jaundice** (a visually detectable buildup of bile pigments in the blood).

Approximately 10% of the white population more than 29 years of age in the United States is estimated to have gallstones. There are basically two types of gallstones, cholesterol stones and pigment stones, although both types have a mixed composition.

In many individuals, the quantity of bile produced by the liver may be normal, but the quality

CLINICAL APPLICATIONS—cont'd

may be abnormal. To be stable, bile must contain certain proportions of bile salts, phospholipids, and cholesterol. If the patient has a relative excess of cholesterol, it may precipitate to form gallstones. Cholesterol stones are 50% to 75% cholesterol, and most contain a pigment center (bilirubin) that probably acted as a nidus for stone formation. Approximately 50% of the bile produced by individuals who do not have gallstones is supersaturated with cholesterol. All bile produced by patients with cholesterol stones is supersaturated with cholesterol. In nonobese patients with cholesterol stones, the amount of lipids in bile is decreased. In obese patients, the amount of cholesterol is increased. In both groups, the bile acid pool is reduced for some reason to about 50% of normal. Supersaturation results in crystal formation and the growth of crystals into stones.

Pigment stones are produced when unconjugated bilirubin precipitates with calcium to form a stone. In normal bile, bilirubin is solubilized by conjugation to glucuronic acid, and approximately only 1% remains unconjugated. Gallbladder bile from patients with pigment stones, however, is saturated with unconjugated bilirubin. The enzyme β-glucuronidase is responsible for the deconjugation of bilirubin within the gallbladder. The enzyme is released from the wall of the damaged gallbladder and is present in high concentrations in a variety of bacteria, including *Escherichia coli*, which may infect the gallbladder. These unconjugated pigments, which are less soluble, then precipitate to form pigment stones or a nidus for precipitation of cholesterol.

Abnormalities of the bile ducts and gallbladder usually are secondary to the processes of obstruction (e.g., stones, tumor) and infection. **Obstruction** can result in severe pain and can lead to reflux of bile into the liver parenchyma and eventually the systemic circulation. Abnormalities of intestinal function can alter the secretion of products that undergo enterohepatic circulation. For example, if the terminal ileum is diseased or removed, bile salt absorption is reduced. This decreases the bile salt pool (and hence bile salt secretion) and increases synthesis of bile acids by the liver. In addition, bile acids that enter the colon induce water secretion by the colonic mucosa and cause diarrhea.

CLINICAL TESTS

The major tests of bile secretion involve measurement of serum levels of endogenous substances normally secreted in the bile, measurement of secretion of exogenous substances injected into the blood, and x-ray, scintigraphic, and ultrasonographic visualizations of the biliary tract.

Plasma levels of both bile salts and bile pigments are elevated in many types of hepatobiliary disease. Of these substances, bilirubin is the most commonly measured entity. Abnormalities in hepatic function often can be detected before the elevation of serum bilirubin and the development of jaundice. This measurement is done by intravenously injecting chemicals such as sulfobromophthalein and indocyanine green. These substances normally are taken up and secreted by the same anionic transport system used for the hepatic secretion of bile pigments. Impairment of hepatocyte function is characterized by a slower than normal disappearance of these injected substances from the blood.

Many **gallstones** are radiopaque and can be visualized on a plain abdominal x-ray film. Others, however, are radiolucent and thus are not obvious; radiopaque dye is required to facilitate visualization of these stones. The dye usually consists of iodinated anions that are taken up and secreted by the anionic transport system of the hepatocytes. The stones are then surrounded by

Continued

CLINICAL TESTS—cont'd

the dye and appear as holes in the contrast medium. Radiopaque dyes are effective only if the anionic transport system of the hepatocytes is functional; therefore, the tests do not work in the presence of jaundice. Scintigraphy and especially ultrasound examination are becoming routine for the confirmation or exclusion of gallstone disease. Ultrasonography can provide information about the thickness of the gallbladder wall, the presence of intramural gas, and even the diameter of the intrahepatic and extrahepatic bile ducts.

SUMMARY

1. Bile is secreted by the liver as a complex mixture of bile acids, phospholipids, cholesterol, bile pigments, electrolytes, and water.
2. Primary bile acids are synthesized from cholesterol by the hepatocytes and are conjugated to taurine and glycine. Conjugated bile acids are amphipathic and, along with phospholipids and cholesterol, form mixed micelles in aqueous solution at pH values found in the intestine. Micelles take part in the digestion and absorption of dietary lipids and lipid-soluble substances.
3. Hepatic bile secretion depends primarily on the secretion of bile acids. Bile acid secretion in turn depends on hepatocyte uptake of bile acids from the portal blood and on bile acid synthesis. Bile secretion depends to a lesser degree on electrolyte secretion by hepatocytes and ductule cells.
4. During the fasting state, most secreted bile is stored in the gallbladder, where electrolytes and water are absorbed, thus concentrating the bile acids as an isosmotic micellar solution. Small amounts of bile empty into the duodenum during the MMC.
5. During the fed state, the gallbladder contracts, thereby expelling larger quantities of bile into the duodenum. Gallbladder contraction mostly results from the action of CCK released from the upper intestine in response to food products.
6. In the intestine, some bile acids are deconjugated, and some primary bile acids are dehydroxylated to form secondary bile acids. These, along with the still-conjugated primary bile acids, are absorbed from the intestine either passively along the length of intestine or actively through an Na^+-coupled transport process in the ileum. Once absorbed into the portal circulation, bile acids are returned to the liver, where they are actively absorbed by an Na^+-coupled transport process, conjugated (if need be), and resecreted. Bile acids lost into the feces are replaced by new synthesis. This pattern of bile acid secretion, absorption, and resecretion is termed the *enterohepatic circulation*.

KEY WORDS AND CONCEPTS

Bile
Bile acids
Micelles
Critical micellar concentration
Phospholipids
Cholesterol
Bile pigments
Inorganic ions
Gallbladder
Enterohepatic circulation
Liver
Hepatocytes
Bilirubin
Hemoglobin
Bile acid–dependent secretion
Bile acid–independent secretion
Bile duct
Sphincter of Oddi
Cholecystokinin
Jaundice
Obstruction
Bacterial infections
Gallstones

SUGGESTED READINGS

Dawson P: Bile formation and the enterohepatic circulation. In Johnson LR, editor: ed 5, *Physiology of the Gastrointestinal Tract*, vol 2, San Diego, 2012, Elsevier.

Mawe GM, Lavoie B, Nelson MT, Pozo MJ: Neuromuscular function in the biliary tract. In Johnson LR, editor: ed 5, *Physiology of the Gastrointestinal Tract*, vol 2, San Diego, 2012, Elsevier.

Moseley RH: Bile secretion. In Yamada T, Alpers DH, Laine L, et al: ed 3, *Textbook of Gastroenterology*, vol 1, Philadelphia, 1999, Lippincott Williams & Wilkins.

Scharschmidt BF: Bilirubin metabolism, bile formation, and gallbladder and bile duct function. In Sleisenger MH, Fordtran JS, editors: ed 5, *Gastrointestinal Disease*, vol 2, Philadelphia, 1993, Saunders.

Wolkoff AW: Mechanisms of hepatocyte organic ion transport. In Johnson LR, editor: ed 5, *Physiology of the Gastrointestinal Tract*, vol 2, San Diego, 2012, Elsevier.

DIGESTION AND ABSORPTION OF NUTRIENTS

- Indicate the sources, types, and functions of the primary digestive enzymes.
- Explain the transport processes and the pathways involved in the absorption of nutrients.
- Describe the processes involved in the digestion and absorption of carbohydrates.
- Indicate problems that may result in the malabsorption of carbohydrates.
- Describe the digestion and absorption of proteins.
- Explain the role of trypsin in protein digestion and how it may be involved in the development of pancreatitis.
- Understand the significance of carriers for dipeptides physiologically and clinically.
- Discuss the processes involved in the digestion and absorption of the various lipids including the roles of micelles and chylomicrons.
- Discuss disorders that may lead to steatorrhea (excessive fat in the stool).

Motility and secretion are regulated to ensure the efficient digestion of food and absorption of nutrients across the mucosa of the gastrointestinal (GI) tract. This chapter explains how food is broken down into small absorbable molecules and how these products are transported into the blood.

STRUCTURAL-FUNCTIONAL ASSOCIATIONS

Food assimilation takes place primarily in the small intestine and is aided by anatomic modifications that increase the luminal surface area—Kerckring's folds, villi, and microvilli. The microvilli are prominent on the apical surface of columnar epithelial cells or enterocytes and occur to a lesser extent on goblet cells. Collectively the microvillous regions constitute the **brush border.**

Several cell types make up the intestinal epithelium. Students of digestive and absorptive physiology are most familiar with **enterocytes** and **goblet cells.** Enterocytes function in digestion, absorption, and secretion. Goblet cells secrete mucus. The function of mucus is not clear but may be related to physical, chemical, and immunologic protection. Both enterocytes and goblet cells are derived from a common stem cell within the intestinal crypts. Enterocytes and goblet cells become differentiated as they move upward from the base of the crypt, and their characteristics are expressed more strongly as they migrate farther up the villus. As they reach the tip of the villus, the cells are extruded and become a component of the succus entericus. Following division of the stem cells, some daughter cells migrate to the base of the crypt where they differentiate into **Paneth cells,** which are part of the mucosal defenses against infection. These cells secrete several agents that destroy bacteria (lysozymes and defensins) or produce inflammatory responses (tumor necrosis factor-α [TNF-α]).

In humans, the time needed to replace the entire population of epithelial cells (the cell turnover time) is 3 to 6 days. Cell proliferation, differentiation, and maturation are influenced by GI hormones, growth factors, other endocrine substances, and the nature of the material in the lumen. These processes are also altered by starvation, irradiation, and the loss of a portion of the bowel. The rapid proliferative rate of the intestinal mucosa makes it vulnerable to radiation and chemotherapy, procedures used to treat cancer. Despite the interplay between a basic dynamic process and the extrinsic factors that affect epithelial development, under normal conditions the mucosal appearance remains relatively constant.

DIGESTION

Digestion is the chemical breakdown of food by enzymes secreted by glandular cells in the mouth, chief cells in the stomach, and the exocrine cells of the pancreas, or enzymes bound to the apical membranes of enterocytes. Although some digestion of carbohydrates, proteins, and fats takes place in the stomach, the final breakdown of these substances occurs in the small intestine.

The enzymes important in digestion are summarized in Figure 11-1. **Luminal** or **cavital digestion** results from enzymes secreted by the salivary glands, stomach, and pancreas. Significant chemical degradation of food is also carried out by hydrolytic enzymes associated with the small intestinal brush border. Hydrolysis by these enzymes is termed **contact** or **membrane digestion**. *Membrane digestion* is a more acceptable term, because *contact digestion* connotes activity by exogenous enzymes that become adsorbed on the epithelial surface. Membrane digestion refers to hydrolysis by enzymes synthesized by epithelial cells and inserted into the apical membrane as integral components. The half-life of membrane-bound enzymes (e.g., oligosaccharidases) is shorter than that of the epithelial cells. Thus breakdown and resynthesis occur several times during the life of a single cell.

Digestion and absorption of essentially all major dietary products take place in the small intestine. Despite the degradation of colonic contents by bacteria, physiologically important digestion does not occur in the colon. Nonetheless, absorption in this organ is impressive. A practical illustration is that some medications administered as rectal suppositories are systemically functional. During periods of health the principal substances absorbed from the colon are water and electrolytes. However, life is possible

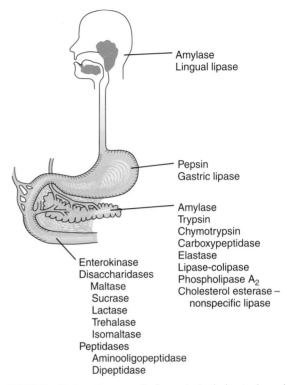

FIGURE 11-1 ■ Source of the principal luminal and membrane-bound digestive enzymes.

without this organ, as evidenced by patients who thrive after colectomy.

ABSORPTION

Although the brush border is the site of activity for a number of digestive enzymes, it is also the barrier that must be traversed by nutrients, water, and electrolytes on the way to the blood or lymph. The terms *transport* and *absorption* often are used interchangeably to mean the movement of materials from the intestinal lumen into the blood. *Secretion* implies movement in the opposite direction.

Mucosal Membrane

Conceptually the plasma membrane of the enterocyte is often considered the only factor restricting the free movement of substances from the gut lumen into the blood or lymph. However, transmural movement actually takes place over a complex pathway. This is

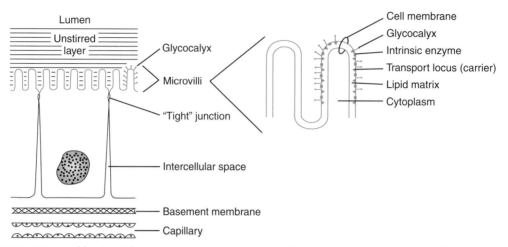

FIGURE 11-2 ■ Mucosal barrier. Solutes moving across the enterocyte from the intestinal lumen to the blood must traverse an unstirred layer of fluid, a glycocalyx, the apical membrane, the cytoplasm of the cell, the basolateral cell membrane, the basement membrane, and finally the wall of the capillary of the lymphatic vessel. Microvilli are morphologic modifications of the cell membrane that comprise the brush border. The importance of this region in the digestion and absorption of nutrients is depicted by the enlarged microvillus, which illustrates the spatial arrangement of enzymes and carrier molecules.

conveyed schematically in Figure 11-2 and includes (1) an **unstirred layer of fluid,** (2) the **glycocalyx** ("fuzzy coat") covering the microvilli, (3) the cell membrane, (4) the cytoplasm of the enterocyte, (5) the basal or lateral cell membrane, (6) the intercellular space, (7) the basement membrane, and (8) the membrane of the capillary or lymph vessel.

Transport Processes

An outstanding property of the enterocyte membrane is its capacity to control the flux of solutes and fluid between the lumen and blood. This process involves several mechanisms. Pinocytosis occurs at the base of microvilli and may be a major mechanism in the uptake of protein. Other uptake processes include **passive diffusion, facilitated diffusion,** and **active transport.** In the case of passive diffusion, the epithelium behaves like an inert barrier, and the particles traverse this cell layer through pores in the cell membrane or through intercellular spaces. Lipid-soluble substances can diffuse through lipid portions of the membrane. The tight junction between apposing enterocytes (see Fig. 11-2) forms a mechanical seal that prevents mixing of interstitial fluid with luminal contents. This seal, however, is relatively leaky to ions and water in certain regions of the intestine, thus allowing some exchange between the lumen and intercellular spaces.

ADAPTATION OF DIGESTIVE AND ABSORPTIVE PROCESSES

Alterations in intestinal functions in response to a variety of factors are well documented. Functional adjustments that maintain homeostasis or allow an animal to cope better with its environment are termed *adaptations.* The quality and degree of adjustment depend on the type of environmental stimulus encountered. Clinical situations in which the capacity to adapt is magnified are small bowel resection and bypass. Until recently physicians knew only that a patient subjected to one of these operations underwent an initial phase of undernutrition, steatorrhea, and acidic diarrhea and that these symptoms tended to be alleviated with time. Relief from the symptoms is believed to be attributable to adaptations. For example, after proximal bowel resection or bypass, the remaining segment undergoes hyperplastic changes accompanied by enhancement of particular absorptive and digestive functions. Adaptation is limited in some circumstances. This point is illustrated by the fact that the carrier-mediated absorption of vitamin B_{12} and bile salts is confined strictly to the terminal ileum. Other regions of the GI tract cannot compensate if the absorptive capacity for these compounds in the ileum is lost.

With certain genetic abnormalities, such as **lactase deficiency,** the capacity to adapt is lost. Lactase deficiency and also pancreatic and intestinal diseases of varied origin contribute to maldigestion and malabsorption.

CARBOHYDRATE ASSIMILATION

Principal Dietary Forms

The average daily intake of carbohydrates, which account for approximately 50% of the calories ingested, is approximately 300 g in the United States. **Starch** comprises approximately 50% of the total, **sucrose** approximately 30%, **lactose** 6%, and **maltose** 1% to 2%. Trehalose, glucose, fructose, sorbitol, cellulose, hemicellulose, and pectins make up most of the remainder. Starch is a high-molecular-weight compound consisting of two polysaccharides, amylose and amylopectin. Amylose is a straight-chain polymer of glucose linked by α-1,4-glycosidic bonds. The repeating disaccharide unit is maltose. **Amylopectin,** a plant starch, is the major form of carbohydrate in the diet and is similar to amylose; however, in addition to 1,4- linkages there is a 1,6- linkage for every 20 to 30 glucose units. Glycogen is a high-molecular-weight polysaccharide similar to amylopectin in molecular structure but having considerably more 1,6-linkages. Maltose and trehalose are dimers of glucose in 1,4- and 1,1- linkages, respectively. Sucrose is a disaccharide consisting of 1 mole (mol) of glucose bound at the number 1 carbon to the number 2 carbon of fructose. Lactose is 1 mol of galactose bound at the number 1 carbon to the number 4 carbon of glucose in a β-linkage.

Digestion

Luminal digestion of starch begins in the mouth with the action of salivary α-amylase and ends in the small intestine through the action of pancreatic α-amylase, which is 94% homologous to salivary amylase. Human salivary and pancreatic amylases have optimum activities near neutral pH and are activated by chloride

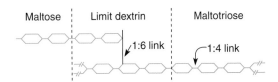

FIGURE 11-3 ■ Products of starch hydrolysis by α-amylase.

(Cl⁻). Although salivary amylase is destroyed by acid in the stomach, some enzymatic activity occurs within a bolus of food while it remains unmixed with acid in the orad stomach. Most starch digestion, however, occurs in the small intestine. Hydrolysis occurs not only in the lumen but also at the surface of epithelial cells because some amylase is adsorbed to the brush border.

Amylase attacks only the interior α-1,4-bonds of amylose, thus yielding maltose and the trisaccharide maltotriose. Hydrolysis of amylopectin and glycogen yields similar products in addition to α-limit dextrins (Fig. 11-3). The latter are oligosaccharides of glucose, formed because the α-1,6- linkages and the α-1,4- bonds near the 1,6- linkages are resistant to amylase. As much as one third of amylopectin cannot be hydrolyzed by amylase. The average α-limit dextrin contains 5 to 10 glucose residues and is rapidly hydrolyzed by membrane-bound enzymes.

Products of amylase action on starch and other major dietary sugars are hydrolyzed by brush border carbohydrases. The process begins with the removal of α-limit dextrins (Fig. 11-4). Glucoamylase is the most active enzyme, but sucrase and isomaltase also cleave these bonds. The glucose residues are removed sequentially from the nonreducing ends until a 1-6 branch point is reached. This bond is hydrolyzed by isomaltase, which also is called α-dextrinase. Sucrase cleaves 100% of sucrose to yield glucose and fructose. All lactose is broken down into glucose and galactose by lactase. Trehalase breaks the α-1,1- bonds of trehalose into glucose. Sucrase, lactase, and trehalase break down sucrose, lactose, and trehalose, respectively. Thus the only products of sugar digestion are glucose, galactose, and fructose.

Sucrase and isomaltase occur together as a molecular complex. The finding that congenital deficiencies of sucrase and α-dextrinase occur together reveals a close functional relationship between these two enzymes. In humans, sucrase-isomaltase is a compound molecule,

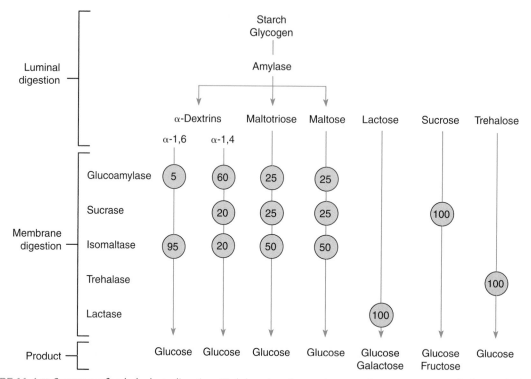

FIGURE 11-4 ■ Summary of carbohydrate digestion. *Circled numbers* denote the approximate percentage of substrate hydrolyzed by a particular brush border enzyme. The same carrier actively transports glucose and galactose into the cell, whereas fructose is absorbed by facilitated diffusion.

one unit with absolute specificity for sucrose and one for the α-1,6- linkage of an α-limit dextrin.

In general the small intestine has a large disacchari-dase reserve, so much that the rate-limiting step in sugar assimilation is not digestion but the absorption of free hexoses following hydrolysis. Under normal circumstances the major portion of sugar assimilation is complete in the proximal jejunum. The human GI tract does not possess cellulase capable of digesting the β-glucose bonds of cellulose and hemicellulose. These carbohydrates account for the undigestible fiber present in the diet.

Absorption of Digestion Products

For the body to use food-derived monosaccharides, they must be absorbed. Figure 11-5 shows how glucose absorption from the intestine occurs by passive as well as active processes. Although aqueous channels are present between enterocytes and pores in brush border membranes, dietary hexoses are too large to

penetrate the membranes in any significant degree by passive diffusion. In humans, the major routes of absorption are via three membrane carrier systems: SGLT-1, GLUT-5, and GLUT-2.

Fructose is transported by facilitated diffusion. The carrier involved is GLUT-5, which is located in the apical membrane of the enterocyte. The transport process does not depend on either sodium (Na^+) or energy. Fructose exits the basolateral membrane by another facilitated diffusion process involving the GLUT-2 transporter. GLUT-2 also is responsible for the exit of glucose and galactose from the absorbing cell.

The carrier systems for fructose and glucose and/or galactose differ insofar as the fructose carrier cannot be energized for active transport, whereas the glucose carrier can. Glucose and galactose are absorbed by secondary active transport via an Na^+-dependent carrier system (SGLT-1) (Fig. 11-6). Mutual inhibition of glucose or galactose transport by the presence of the other indicates that they are transported by a common carrier.

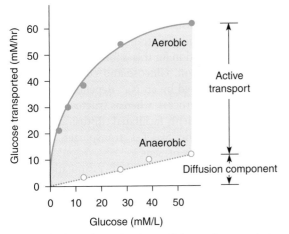

FIGURE 11-5 ■ Absorption rates of glucose from a solution perfused through the intestine of a guinea pig. In the absence of oxygen, the rate of mediated uptake is proportional to concentration. When oxygen is available for cellular respiration, the uptake is greater, and the carrier system can be energized for active transport. mM/L, millimoles/liter; mM/hr, micromoles/hour. (*Modified from Ricklis E, Quastel JH: Effects of cations on sugar absorption by isolated surviving guinea pig intestine. Can J Biochem Physiol 36:348-362, 1958.*)

The glucose entry step depicted in Figure 11-6 involves a carrier that binds Na^+ and galactose or glucose molecules; 2 Na^+ for each glucose or galactose molecule are transported into the cell. The entry step is only slightly reversible because of removal of intracellular Na^+ by the pump on the basolateral membrane. Energy input (adenosine triphosphate [ATP]) drives the Na^+ pump and maintains an Na^+ gradient favoring glucose entry. Inhibition of the Na^+, potassium (K^+)-ATPase with specific chemicals (such as ouabain) or interference of cellular energy production leads to cytosolic accumulation of Na^+ and the abolition of active sugar transport. The exit of glucose from the cytosol into the intracellular space is attributed partly to diffusion but mostly to facilitated diffusion via an Na^+-independent carrier located at the basolateral membrane; this carrier has specificity for all three hexoses (GLUT-2).

Regulation of Absorption

The capacity of the human small intestine to absorb free sugars is enormous. It has been estimated that

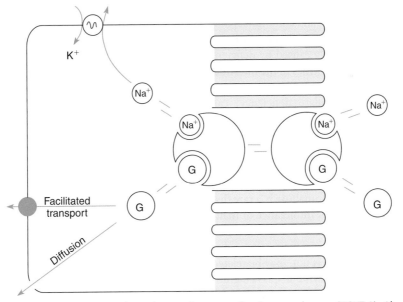

FIGURE 11-6 ■ Summary of a sodium (Na^+)-dependent carrier system for glucose-galactose (SGLT-1). Absorption involves the rapid movement from lumen to blood by an entry step and exit step mediated by two separate carrier molecules with specificity for hexose. The system is energized by an adenosine (ATP)-dependent Na^+ pump that maintains an Na^+ gradient favoring the entry of 2 Na^+ into the cell, with the concomitant cotransport of glucose or galactose (G). When Na^+ is pumped from the cell, more Na^+ and glucose are transported into the cell from the lumen. A carrier (GLUT-2) in the basolateral membrane facilitates the exit of fructose, as well as glucose and galactose, from the cell. The transport capacity of GLUT-2 appears to equal that involved in hexose entry, because hexose does not accumulate within the cells to a significant degree. K^+, potassium.

hexoses equivalent to 22 pounds of sucrose can be absorbed daily. There appears to be little physiologic control of sugar absorption. However, chemoreceptors and osmoreceptors in the proximal small intestine control the motility and emptying of the stomach through a negative feedback process mediated by hormones and neural reflexes. As an example, a volume of isotonic citrate solution of 750 mL that is placed in the human stomach passes into the small bowel in 20 minutes. The volume delivered in the same time is reduced if sucrose or glucose is added to the citrate solution. The amount delivered is related inversely to the sugar concentration.

Abnormalities in Carbohydrate Assimilation

It is obvious from the foregoing considerations that polysaccharides and oligosaccharides are absorbed as monosaccharides. Carbohydrates remaining in the intestinal lumen increase the osmotic pressure of the luminal contents because of defects in digestion and absorption. Bacterial fermentation of these carbohydrates in the lower small intestine and colon adds to this osmotic effect. The osmotic retention of water in the lumen leads to diarrhea, bloating, and abdominal pain.

Diarrhea caused by the poor assimilation of dietary carbohydrates is most commonly caused by deficiencies in carbohydrate-splitting enzymes in the intestinal brush border. **Lactase deficiency,** the most frequently observed congenital disaccharidase deficiency, can exist in the absence of any other intestinal malfunction. The inability to digest lactose is actually a developmental change. In fact, a large percentage of the individuals of most races, other than those originating in Northern Europe, will lose lactase activity later in life. Intolerance of sucrose and isomaltose is a rare disease found primarily in children. Intolerance of maltose has not been documented. The observation that lactase deficiency is a relatively common genetic disease, whereas maltase deficiency is not, may be related to the finding that only one enzyme displays significant lactase activity, although several display activity against maltose (see Fig. 11-4). Thus maltose intolerance would require the simultaneous absence of all enzymes possessing maltase activity. Maldigestion of starch in humans is nonexistent because pancreatic amylase is secreted in tremendous excess.

Intolerance to glucose and galactose has been documented in rare instances. In these cases the patients thrive and show no symptoms when they are fed fructose. The explanation for this is found in the specificity of sugar absorption. Glucose and chemically related sugars are absorbed by an Na^+-dependent secondary active transport process, whereas fructose is absorbed by Na^+-independent facilitated diffusion. Thus in these patients, the SGLT-1 transporter is absent, whereas GLUT-5 is present.

Besides defects in carbohydrate assimilation caused by the congenital or acquired enzyme deficiencies, assimilation of dietary sugars may be impaired by diseases of the GI tract. Celiac disease, certain bacterial infections, and some protozoan and helminth infections are associated with inflammation and structural derangements in the small bowel mucosa. These conditions are often attended by brush border enzyme deficiencies and hexose malabsorption (Fig. 11-7). It is not uncommon to find lactase deficiency as a long-term consequence of intestinal disease because this enzyme is present in the intestine at low levels compared with maltase and sucrase.

Symptoms of osmotic diarrhea include cramps and abdominal distention. An oral tolerance test can be used to diagnose disaccharidase deficiency if this is a suspected cause. After an overnight fast, adult patients are fed 50 g of lactose in a 10% aqueous solution (children are usually fed 2 g/kg of body weight). Blood

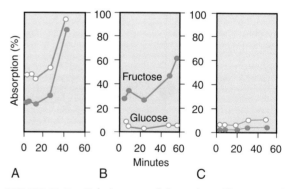

FIGURE 11-7 ■ Relative rates of absorption of fructose and glucose in an equimolar mixture studied by an intubation technique in a control subject **(A)**, a patient with glucose malabsorption **(B)**, and a patient with celiac disease **(C)**. *(From Dahlquist A: In Sipple HL, McNutt KW (eds): Sugars in Nutrition. New York, Academic Press, 1974.)*

samples are taken for glucose analysis before and at 5, 10, 15, 30, 45, and 60 minutes after lactose administration. An increase in blood glucose of at least 25 mg/dL over fasted levels indicates normal hydrolysis of lactose and normal absorption of the glucose product. A flat lactose tolerance curve or failure to observe a rise in blood glucose to more than 25 mg/dL following lactose ingestion indicates low lactase activity. A value between 20 and 25 mg/dL is questionable. In this case the test may be repeated or, if laboratory facilities permit, intestinal biopsy specimens can be collected and examined for enzyme activity. In dealing with biopsy specimens, enzyme activity usually is expressed as units per gram of tissue protein. Tolerance tests for disaccharides other than lactose are seldom performed, but a similar procedure would suffice. Glucose or galactose tolerance tests should be performed to exclude monosaccharide malabsorption as the cause of a flat lactose tolerance curve.

PROTEIN ASSIMILATION

Digestion

The daily dietary intake of protein varies considerably in different parts of the world. People from Eastern countries, who eat a high-carbohydrate diet in the form of rice, consume less protein than those from meat-eating Western societies, where a typical diet contains more than 100 g per day. Secretions from the salivary glands, stomach, pancreas, and intestines along with sloughed cells add another 40 g protein per day, which is digested and absorbed in the same manner as dietary protein.

Protein digestion begins in the stomach with the action of pepsin. The enzyme precursor pepsinogen is secreted by chief cells in response to a meal and low gastric pH. Acid in the stomach is responsible for activating pepsinogen to pepsin. Three pepsin isozymes have been recognized. All have a pH optimum of 1 to 3 and are denatured above pH 5. Pepsin is an endopeptidase with specificity for peptide bonds involving aromatic L-amino acids.

Pepsin activity terminates when the gastric contents mix with alkaline pancreatic juice in the small bowel. Chyme in the intestine stimulates the release of secretin and cholecystokinin (CCK), which in turn, along

with cholinergic nerve activity, cause the pancreas to secrete bicarbonate and enzymes into the intestinal lumen.

The two general classes of pancreatic proteases are **endopeptidases** and **exopeptidases.** The basis of classification and the particular characteristics of specific enzymes belonging to each class are given in Table 11-1.

Pancreatic proteases are secreted into the duodenum as inactive precursors. **Trypsinogen,** which lacks proteolytic activity, is activated by **enterokinase,** an enzyme located on the brush border of duodenal enterocytes. The exact chemical composition of enterokinase is not known; however, the fact that the molecule is 41% carbohydrate probably prevents its rapid digestion by proteolytic enzymes. The activity of enterokinase is stimulated by trypsinogen, and it is released from the brush border membrane by bile salts. Enterokinase activates trypsinogen by releasing a hexapeptide from the N-terminal end of the precursor molecule (Fig. 11-8). Active trypsin, once formed, acts autocatalytically in the manner of enterokinase to activate the bulk of trypsinogen. Trypsin also activates other peptidase precursors

TABLE 11-1	
Principal Pancreatic Proteases	
Enzyme	*Primary Action*
Endopeptidases	Hydrolyze interior peptide bonds of polypeptides and proteins
Trypsin	Attacks peptide bonds involving basic amino acids; yields products with basic amino acids at C-terminal end
Chymotrypsin	Attacks peptide bonds involving aromatic amino acids, leucine, glutamine, and methionine; yields peptide products with these amino acids at C-terminal end
Elastase	Attacks peptide bonds involving neutral aliphatic amino acids; yields products with neutral amino acids at C-terminal end
Exopeptidases	Hydrolyze external peptide bonds of polypeptides and protein
Carboxypeptidase A	Attacks peptides with aromatic and neutral aliphatic amino acids at C-terminal end
Carboxypeptidase B	Attacks peptides with basic amino acids at C-terminal end

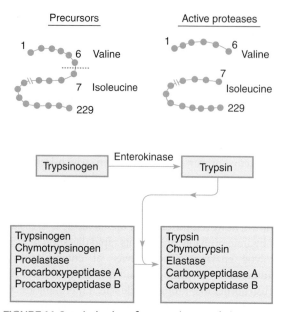

1   6   Valine

1   6   Valine

7

7   Isoleucine

Isoleucine

229

229

Trypsinogen   Enterokinase   Trypsin

Trypsinogen	Trypsin
Chymotrypsinogen	Chymotrypsin
Proelastase	Elastase
Procarboxypeptidase A	Carboxypeptidase A
Procarboxypeptidase B	Carboxypeptidase B

FIGURE 11-8 ■ Activation of pancreatic proteolytic enzymes. The process begins in the lumen when enterokinase cleaves a hexapeptide from trypsinogen and converts it to the active enzyme trypsin.

from the pancreas (see Fig. 11-8). **Chymotrypsinogen** is activated by cleavage of the peptide bond between arginine and isoleucine, which are the fifteenth and sixteenth amino acid residues at the N-terminus. Although structural rearrangement occurs, no peptide fragment is released because of a disulfide bond between the cysteine residues at positions 1 and 122 in the protein chain. This configuration is the active form of chymotrypsinogen. Cleavage at other points in the chymotrypsinogen molecule produces other molecular species of chymotrypsin having relatively little physiologic importance. The exact mechanism for activation of **proelastase** is not known, and activation of **procarboxypeptidases A and B** is relatively complicated, involving proteolysis of at least two proenzymes.

Once in the small intestine, pancreatic enzymes undergo rapid inactivation because of autodigestion. Trypsin is the enzyme primarily responsible for inactivation.

Development of Pancreatitis

In developed countries, 80% of the cases of acute pancreatitis are the result of either biliary stone disease or ethanol abuse. Alcohol consumption is the major cause of chronic pancreatitis.

As pointed out previously, trypsin plays a central role in the activation of other pancreatic zymogens. Normally trypsin remains as inactive trypsinogen until it is secreted into the duodenal lumen. The mechanisms responsible for the intracellular activation of trypsin are not totally clear. One hypothesis states that it is catalyzed by lysosomal hydrolases after the colocalization of these hydrolases with digestive zymogens within membrane-bound organelles during the early stages of pancreatitis.

Premature activation of trypsinogen within the pancreas initiates the entire activation cascade of other proteases, results in autodigestion of pancreatic cells, and causes acute pancreatitis. The body has several mechanisms to prevent premature trypsin activation. These include synthesis of pancreatic trypsin inhibitors, isolation of zymogens from lysosomes, and a site on trypsin that is susceptible to digestion by trypsin itself. Thus when trypsin comes into contact with other trypsin molecules, it is able to cleave them and irreversibly inactivate the enzyme.

This site for autodigestion is an arginine residue in position 117. Research has located a single guanine-to-adenine gene mutation that results in the substitution of histidine for arginine (R117H). This substitution prevents trypsin from being inactivated and was discovered in several families of patients with hereditary pancreatitis. Thus this mutation eliminates one of the failsafe mechanisms preventing the premature activation of trypsinogen and is the basis for at least one form of hereditary pancreatitis.

Absorption of Digestion Products

Membrane digestion and absorption are closely related phenomena in protein assimilation, and physiologists have been occupied by two fundamental questions concerning them: (1) In what form do products of proteolysis cross the brush border membrane of the epithelial cell? (2) In what form do these products leave the cell to enter the blood?

L-Isomers of some amino acids are absorbed by carrier-mediated mechanisms in much the same manner as glucose is absorbed. As with glucose, the cell entry process requires Na^+ as part of a ternary complex (see Fig. 11-6), and uphill transfer occurs by secondary

TABLE 11-2

Carrier Systems for the Transport of Amino Acids

Transport System	Substrate	Dependence on Sodium Gradient
Brush Border Membrane		
B⁰	Neutral L-amino acids	Yes
B⁰,ᵗ	Neutral L- and cationic L-amino acids	Yes
b⁰,ᵗ	Neutral L- and cationic amino acids, cystine	No
IMINO	Imino acids	Yes
B	Taurine, β-alanine	Yes
X⁻ᴬᴳ	Anionic amino acids	Yes
ASC	Neutral L-amino acids	Yes
N	Glutamine, asparagine histidine	Yes
PAT	Small neutral amino acids	No
Basolateral Membrane		
A	Neutral L-amino acids	Yes
GLY	Glycine	Yes
Y+	Cationic amino acids	No
L	Neutral L-amino acids	No
Y+L	Neutral L-amino acids, cationic amino acids	Yes/no
ASC	Small L- and D-amino acids	No

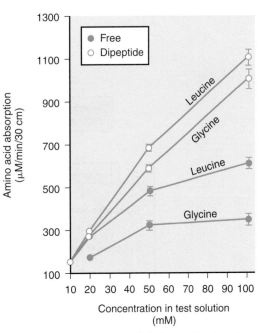

FIGURE 11-9 ■ Jejunal rates of glycine and leucine absorption (mean ± SEM, five subjects) from perfusion of test solutions containing either L-glycyl-L-leucine or an equimolar mixture of free L-glycine and free L-leucine. *(From Adibi SA: Intestinal transport of dipeptides in man: relative importance of hydrolysis and intact absorption. J Clin Invest 50:2266-2275, 1971.)*

active transport. Other amino acids and some of those absorbed by active transport can also be absorbed by facilitated diffusion processes that do not require Na⁺ (Table 11-2). A new class of electrogenic *proton-dependent amino acid transporters*—PAT proteins—has been cloned. Present on the apical membrane, PAT proteins transport short-chain amino acids (glycine, alanine, serine, proline) into the cell, along with a hydrogen ion (H⁺). Thus the entry of the amino acid is coupled with the movement of a proton down its electrochemical gradient.

Certain L-amino acids compete with one another for uptake by intestinal cells. Studies of competition have led to the recognition of several different carrier systems for amino acid absorption (see Table 11-2). There is little doubt that the absorption of free amino acids by gut mucosa is physiologically important. However, amino acids appear in portal blood faster and reach a higher level when peptides from an acid hydrolysate of protein contact the gut mucosa than

when there is an equimolar solution of free amino acids (Fig. 11-9). Moreover, greater amounts of total nitrogen are absorbed from a solution of trypsin hydrolysate of proteins than from an equivalent solution of amino acids in free form. Competition for transport between two chemically related amino acids is not observed when the same two acids are absorbed after ingestion of their dipeptides and tripeptides. In addition, the site in the intestine for the maximum absorption of amino acids in small peptide form is different from that for the absorption of free amino acids. The absorptive capacity for dipeptides and tripeptides is greater in the proximal intestine, whereas the capacity for absorbing single amino acids is greater in the distal intestine. The current explanation of these findings is that a separate carrier system for small peptides is involved in absorption. For example, free glycine absorption requires an amino acid carrier system. If saturation of the system occurs under physiologic conditions, the maximum rate of uptake becomes

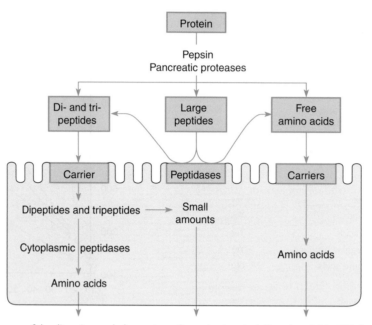

FIGURE 11-10 ■ Summary of the digestion and absorption of protein. Luminal digestion yields 20% free amino acids and 80% peptides consisting primarily of two to six amino acid residues.

limiting. If, however, a second carrier for dipeptides or tripeptides of glycine is present, the amino acids can enter the cell in small peptide form. Thus two separate systems for glycine entry exist and work in a parallel manner.

The prevailing concepts regarding protein assimilation are illustrated in Figure 11-10. Luminal digestion of a protein meal produces approximately 20% free amino acids and 80% small peptides. As with the free acids, dipeptides and tripeptides resulting from digestion can be absorbed intact by a carrier-mediated process. However, tetrapeptides, pentapeptides, and hexapeptides are poorly absorbed; instead they are hydrolyzed by brush border peptidases to free amino acids or smaller absorbable peptides. Small peptides are absorbed by a carrier with broad specificity. This transport process is independent of the Na^+ gradient and is stimulated by an inwardly directed H^+ gradient. The acidic microclimate pH that normally exists on the luminal surface of the brush border membrane provides the driving force for the peptide transport system. This is referred to as the H^+/peptide cotransporter (PEPT1), and it is functionally coupled to the Na^+/H^+ exchanger, NHE3, in the same membrane.

Peptides that enter enterocytes are hydrolyzed by cytoplasmic peptidases to amino acids. These, in turn, diffuse or are moved by carrier-mediated processes from the intracellular compartment, across the basolateral membrane, into the blood. As is the case with the apical membrane, several different carriers exist in the basolateral membrane (see Table 11-2). Some of these also are Na^+ dependent. A few peptides enter the blood intact, and this may explain why certain biologically active peptides exert their effects when they are given orally.

Abnormalities in Protein Assimilation

Pancreatic insufficiency caused by various diseases, including cystic fibrosis and hereditary pancreatitis, may be associated with a decrease or absence of trypsin and may lead to poor digestion of protein. Cases of primary proteinase deficiency caused by congenital trypsinogen deficiency have been reported. In those patients, chymotrypsin and carboxypeptidase activities are lacking also, because trypsin cannot be formed to activate the precursors of these pancreatic proteases.

Intestinal malabsorption and the failure to reabsorb certain amino acids in the proximal renal tubule

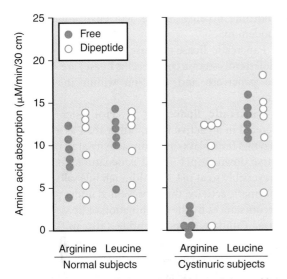

FIGURE 11-11 ■ Jejunal absorption of free arginine and leucine during perfusion of solutions containing L-arginine (1 mM) and L-leucine (1 mM) or L-arginyl-L-leucine (1 mM). Results are from studies carried out in six normal subjects and six cystinuric patients. *(From Silk DBA, Dawson AM. In Crane RK, Guyton AC (eds): International Review of Physiology. III: Gastrointestinal Physiology. Baltimore, University Park Press, 1979.)*

occurs in some hereditary diseases, thus providing evidence that the carriers are identical in the two tissues. **Cystinuria** is characterized by defective transport of the cationic amino acids (arginine, lysine, and ornithine) and cystine in the kidney and the small bowel (Fig. 11-11). The intestinal malabsorptive condition is of little or no consequence in the disability produced by cystinuria, given that the affected amino acids are absorbed as small peptides. However, the disease is severe because cystine has low solubility in water, and as the urine is concentrated in the distal nephron, cystine precipitates and forms stones. **Hartnup's disease** is a hereditary condition in which the active transport of neutral amino acids is deficient in both the renal tubule and the small intestine. An interesting finding is that, although neutral amino acids are not absorbed, they readily appear in the blood after ingestion of their dipeptides. This is compelling evidence that absorption of the dipeptides of certain amino acids is the result of a completely separate process from the one involved in the transport of free amino acids. These patients lose significant amounts of amino acids in their urine, and the condition may become significant in those whose dietary protein intake is low. Because tryptophan is a neutral amino acid, patients with Hartnup's disease suffer from niacin deficiency (pellagra); approximately 50% of the vitamin is synthesized from this amino acid. Tryptophan is also the precursor for the neurotransmitter serotonin, and its decreased synthesis may contribute to the neurologic symptoms associated with this disease.

LIPID ASSIMILATION

Dietary fats comprise the most concentrated source of calories ingested by humans, and intake varies considerably in different cultures depending on the proportion of meat in the diet. Dietary lipids include such substances as triacylglycerides, fat-soluble vitamins (A, D, E, and K), **phospholipids, sterols,** hydrocarbons, and waxes that compose cell walls or membranes of plants and/or animals. The principles of lipid assimilation are dealt with through a consideration of triglycerides, phospholipids, and sterols. The propensity of lipids to form ester linkages and the insolubility of lipids in water make their digestion and absorption a complex process. Unlike carbohydrates and proteins, lipids enter epithelial cells by a sequence of chemical and physical steps that render water-insoluble molecules capable of being absorbed by passive diffusion. The process depends on four major events: (1) secretion of bile and various lipases, (2) emulsification, (3) enzymatic hydrolysis of ester linkages, and (4) the solubilization of lipolytic products within bile salt micelles.

Digestion

Fat assimilation begins in the stomach, where food (partially digested by pepsin) is churned into a coarse mixture and is released in small portions into the duodenum. Except for short-chain fatty acids, no absorption of fat from the stomach occurs. A process, controlled through the action of CCK, slows gastric motility and emptying when fat is in the small intestine. CCK also stimulates the pancreas to secrete lipase and causes contraction of the gallbladder. One function of bile salts released into the duodenum is to perpetuate the **emulsification** of fat droplets by decreasing the surface tension at the oil-water interface. An emulsification is a suspension of fat droplets held apart by phosphatidylcholine (lecithin), bile salts, fatty acids, and other emulsifying agents. The emulsified fat droplets are approximately 1 micrometer (μm) in diameter. The emulsification process is important to increase the surface area of lipids in preparation for their enzymatic hydrolysis and is begun by the churning action of the stomach, which breaks contents into small droplets.

Enzymes from three sources are involved in the digestion of dietary lipids. These enzymes are food-bearing lipases, gastric lipase, and pancreatic lipases.

Enzymes that digest dietary lipids can be found in food per se (e.g., acid lipases, phospholipases). These enzymes may function in autodigestion, a process aided by the acid environment of the stomach. Human milk contains a lipase identical in chemical properties to bile salt–stimulated lipase secreted by the pancreas. Known as **carboxyl ester lipase** (CEL), it is active against cholesterol and vitamin A esters. CEL also hydrolyzes glycerol esters of long-chain fatty acids at the physiologic pH of the small bowel. A feature that distinguishes this esterase from well-known pancreatic lipase is that the latter has pronounced specificity for the 1 and 3 ester bonds of **triglycerides,** whereas CEL shows no positional specificity. Despite the lack of a clear functional role, it is presumed that CEL is important to the use of milk lipids in newborn infants, who have a low intestinal bile salt concentration and absorb glycerol and free fatty acids better than monoglycerides. This presumption is compatible with knowledge that CEL is stable between pH 3.5 and 9 and is broken down only slowly by pepsin. Thus most of the enzyme would pass through the infant's stomach without denaturation. The fact that CEL requires bile salts for activation suggests that it is not functional until it reaches the small intestine.

Lipolytic activity in the human stomach is primarily the result of **gastric lipase** secreted by cells of the corpus and fundus. This enzyme has an acidic pH optimum, ranging from 3 to 6. Gastric lipase acts primarily at the outer ester linkages, thus producing fatty acids and diglycerides. Pancreatic lipase is normally produced in great excess, and the absence of gastric lipase would not alter fat digestion. However, the contribution of gastric lipase can be significant in newborns and patients with pancreatic lipase deficiency or inactivation, such as could occur in Zollinger-Ellison syndrome because of the acid environment of the duodenum.

Pancreatic lipase-colipase, phospholipase A_2, and cholesterol esterase (nonspecific lipase) are secreted by the pancrease and function within the intestinal lumen.

Pancreatic lipase, or glycerol ester lipase, is secreted in an active form, rather than as a precursor enzyme. It displays optimum activity at pH 8, remains active down to pH 5, and is denatured at pH 3.5—irreversibly so at pH 2.5. Although bile salts inhibit its enzymatic activity, this is prevented under physiologic circumstances by the combination of lipase with **colipase.** Colipase, a polypeptide (102 to 107 amino acids) secreted by the pancreas along with lipase in a 1:1 ratio, is secreted as procolipase that is activated when hydrolyzed by trypsin to a peptide containing 96 amino acids. Whereas lipase-colipase complexes are scarce within the duodenum during fasting, the presence of fat stimulates the secretion of these components in large quantities. The inactivation of lipase by bile salts results from the capacity of bile salts to displace lipase at the fat droplet–water interface, where it must exert its action. Colipase prevents inactivation by anchoring lipase to the oil-water interface in the presence of bile salts. Once colipase attaches to the fat droplet, lipase binds to a specific site on the colipase molecule in a 1:1 ratio and consequently carries out its catalytic function, breaking down triglycerides. Colipase also has the capacity to bind to a bile salt micelle. Therefore, the products of fat hydrolysis need diffuse only a short distance to a micelle. Thus, despite its name, colipase has no enzymatic activity of its own.

Lipase is secreted in large excess and rapidly hydrolyzes triglycerides. The enzyme shows positional specificity. It cleaves the 1 and 3 ester linkages, yielding free fatty acids and 2-monoglycerides. That only small amounts of free glycerol are produced reflects the lack of action against the 2 ester linkages (Fig. 11-12).

Phospholipase A_2 is secreted as a proenzyme and is activated by trypsin in much the same fashion as trypsinogen is converted to its active form (i.e., through cleavage of several amino acids from the N-terminus). Bile salts and phospholipids form mixed micelles that become substrates for phospholipase A_2. The enzyme requires bile salts for optimal activity in hydrolyzing

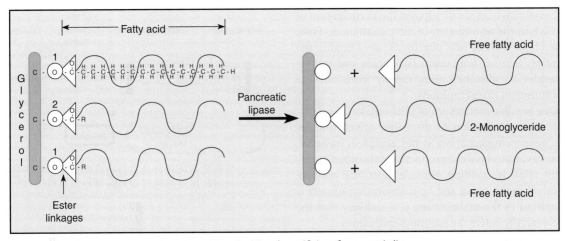

FIGURE 11-12 ■ Positional specificity of pancreatic lipase.

dietary phospholipids at the 2 position and producing lysophospholipid and free fatty acids.

Human pancreatic **cholesterol esterase** hydrolyzes not only cholesterol esters but also the esters of vitamins A, D, and E and those of glycerides. In contrast with pancreatic lipase, cholesterol esterase hydrolyzes all three ester linkages of triglycerides. This capacity accounts for its name—**nonspecific esterase.** Cholesterol esterase is active against substrates that have been incorporated into bile salt micelles. Activity apparently depends on the presence of specific bile salts. The enzyme in humans attacks cholesterol ester in the presence of taurocholate and taurochenodeoxycholate and is probably identical to CEL (previously discussed).

Absorption of Lipolytic Products

In addition to the function just mentioned, bile salts perform an important function in the actual absorption of lipolytic products. Sodium glycocholic and taurocholic acids, which are major bile salts, have both hydrophobic and hydrophilic portions. When their concentration in the intestine is raised to a critical level, bile salt monomers form water-soluble aggregates called **micelles.** The concentration of bile salt at which molecular aggregation occurs is referred to as the **critical micellar concentration.** Conjugated bile salts have a lower critical micellar concentration than do unconjugated bile salts. Whereas emulsion particles are 2000 to 50,000 angstroms (Å) in diameter, mixed micelles are approximately 30 to 100 Å in diameter,

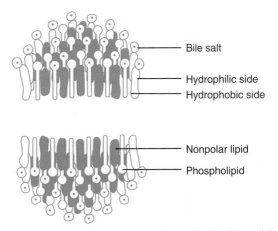

FIGURE 11-13 ■ Solubilization of nonpolar lipid by a bile acid–polar lipid micelle. *(Modified from Hoffman AF, French A, Littman A: Syllabus: Digestion and Absorption. Chicago, American Medical Association, 1975.)*

with a hydrophilic outer surface and a hydrophobic center. In addition, although emulsion particles form a suspension, micelles are in true solution. The water-insoluble monoglycerides from lipolysis are solubilized within the hydrophobic center of the micelle (Fig. 11-13). In turn, fatty acids, lysophospholipids, cholesterol, and fat-soluble vitamins may be solubilized. A mixed micellar solution is water clear. Micellar solubilization is important because it enhances the diffusion of poorly soluble dietary lipids through the unstirred aqueous layer overlying the enterocytes.

Two forms of evidence support the participation of micelles in the assimilation of fatty substances. First, mixed micelles (bile salts plus lipids) are found in the intestine. Second, long-chain fatty acids and monoglycerides are absorbed more rapidly from micellar solutions than from emulsions.

One possible mechanism of lipid uptake by enterocytes is the absorption of the entire mixed micelle. This proposed mechanism is not accepted, however, because various lipolytic products are absorbed at different rates. In addition, because most bile salts are absorbed in the ileum and lipid absorption usually is completed in the midjejunum, it is unlikely that the whole micelle enters the intestinal epithelium.

The importance of micellar solubilization lies in the ability of micelles to diffuse across the unstirred water layer and present large amounts of fatty acids and monoglycerides to the apical membrane of the enterocyte. The brush border membrane is separated from the bulk solution in the intestinal lumen by the unstirred water layer. Single fatty acid and monoglyceride molecules, being poorly soluble in water, move slowly through this barrier. Because uptake depends on the number of molecules in contact with the enterocyte membrane, their absorption is diffusion limited. By contrast, micelles are water soluble, diffuse readily through the unstirred layer, and increase the concentration of fatty acids and monoglycerides at the membrane by 100- to 1000-fold. An acidic microclimate exists next to the plasma membrane that protonates fatty acids, thereby assisting in their release from the micelle and promoting their flux across the apical membrane. Thus mixed micelles keep the intestinal water layer saturated with fatty acids, and absorption proceeds at an optimal rate. Short- and medium-chain fatty acids do not depend on micelles for uptake because of their higher solubility in and diffusion through the unstirred aqueous layer.

Until recently, it was thought that all fat digestion products were absorbed by simple diffusion. However, current evidence indicates a carrier protein-dependent process. Some products such as linoleate show saturable uptake. Uptake in some cases exhibits a specificity that cannot be explained by simple diffusion. The relative contribution of the protein mediated component to total uptake by enterocytes is unclear and is likely to be small.

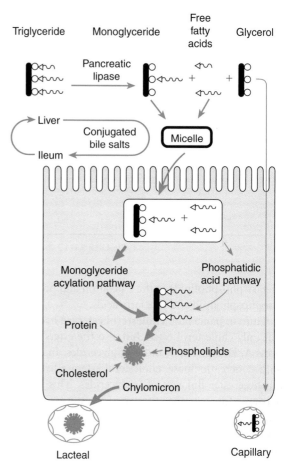

FIGURE 11-14 ■ Summary of the digestion and absorption of triglyceride. Monoglycerides and long-chain fatty acids enter the cells after first being incorporated into micelles. Glycerol and short- and medium-chain acids, because of their solubility in the aqueous unstirred layer, enter without micelle solubilization.

Intracellular Events

Monoglycerides and free fatty acids absorbed by enterocytes are resynthesized into triglycerides by two different pathways: the major pathway, monoglyceride acylation, and the minor pathway, phosphatidic acid acylation (Fig. 11-14).

Monoglyceride Acylation Pathway

The monoglyceride acylation pathway involves the synthesis of triglycerides from 2-monoglycerides and coenzyme A (CoA)-activated fatty acids. Acyl-CoA synthetase is the enzyme that acylates fatty acids. The enzymes monoglyceride and diglyceride acyltransferases are responsible for catalyzing the formation of diglycerides and triglycerides, respectively. The enzymes involved in this pathway are associated mainly with the smooth endoplasmic reticulum.

An interesting aspect of intracellular triglyceride synthesis is that certain fatty acids are used in preference to others. This occurs despite similar rates of absorption by enterocytes and similar rates of enzymatic CoA activation and glyceride esterification. These observations have been explained by the presence of intracellular **fatty acid–binding proteins** (FABPs), which have affinities for fatty acids of different chain lengths and varying degrees of saturation. Such proteins exert their influence after absorption occurs and before esterification takes place.

A current theory on how FABPs operate presumes that absorbed fatty acids bind strongly to the apical membrane of enterocytes. Solubilization is brought about when the fatty acids bind specifically with receptors on FABPs. This facilitates the transfer of the free fatty acids from the apical membrane to the smooth endoplasmic reticulum, where esterification into diglycerides and triglycerides takes place. This process is particularly effective in the intracellular transfer of long-chain fatty acids. By binding long-chain fatty acids and 2-monoglycerides, FABPs maintain the concentration gradient for diffusion of these molecules into the membrane and protect the cell from high concentrations of fatty acids that would be capable of solubilizing lipid membranes. Such a situation could occur during the digestion of a lipid meal. Short- and medium-chain fatty acids, which show less affinity for the cell membrane, are water soluble and not bound by specific proteins. Instead they leave the cell in free form and enter the blood directly, rather than as reesterified triglyceride in chylomicrons.

Phosphatidic Acid Pathway

Triglycerides also can be synthesized from CoA-activated fatty acids and α-glycerophosphate. The latter is formed from phosphorylated glycerol or from the reduction of dihydroxyacetone phosphate derived from glycolysis. One mole of α-glycerophosphate acylated with 2 mol of CoA–fatty acids yields phosphatidic acid, which is dephosphorylated to form diglyceride, which in turn is acylated to form triglyceride. This minor pathway for triglyceride synthesis in the intestine is termed the *phosphatidic acid pathway.*

Phosphatidic acid may also be important in the synthesis of phospholipids such as phosphatidyl choline, ethanolamine, and serine. Alternatively, phospholipids can be derived from acylation of absorbed lysophospholipids by appropriate acyltransferases. The acylation of lysophosphatidyl choline forms phosphatidyl choline, which is used in the formation of chylomicrons.

Dietary cholesterol is absorbed in free form. However, a major fraction leaves the epithelial cells in chylomicrons as esters of fatty acids. This finding is indicative of the highly active intracellular reesterification process. The ratio of free to esterified cholesterol in intestinal lymph is influenced by the amount of cholesterol in the diet (low dietary cholesterol favors the cellular exit of greater amounts of free sterol in chylomicrons). In humans the percentage of net cholesterol absorption decreases as the dietary content increases.

Chylomicrons are lipoprotein particles approximately 750 to 5000 Å in diameter that are synthesized within enterocytes and exist in the form of an emulsion. Although their chemical composition may vary slightly depending on size, chylomicrons are approximately 80% to 90% triglycerides, 8% to 9% phospholipids, 2% cholesterol, 2% protein, and traces of carbohydrate. Studies suggest how triglycerides and esterified cholesterol and fat-soluble vitamins (which form the core) become coated with **apolipoprotein,** phospholipid, and free cholesterol (which make up the surface of the chylomicron). Synthesis of the chylomicron appears to be a two-step process. Small particles containing apolipoprotein B and a small mass of core lipids are synthesized in the rough endoplasmic reticulum. Microsomal triglyceride transfer protein (MTP) is responsible for adding lipids to apolipoprotein B. Concurrently, triglyceride-rich particles that lack apolipoprotein B are synthesized in the lumen of the smooth endoplasmic reticulum. The two particles join, forming a nascent chylomicron, also called a pre-chylomicron. This complex is too large to cross the membrane of the smooth endoplasmic reticulum. This is accomplished by a specialized endoplasmic reticulum–to-Golgi transport vesicle called the pre-chylomicron transport vesicle (PCTV). Following transport to the Golgi apparatus, the prechylomicron acquires apolipoprotein A1 and is glycosylated. The newly formed chylomicrons are secreted by exocytosis into the interstitial space and enter the gaps between the endothelial cells that make up the lacteals. Chylomicrons are too large to enter the pores of blood capillaries.

It is evident that apolipoprotein synthesis by epithelial cells and its incorporation into chylomicrons are essential for fat absorption. Inhibition of protein synthesis causes large amounts of triglyceride to accumulate intracellularly. Several apolipoproteins—termed A, B, C, and E—have been identified in intestinal lymph. Apolipoprotein B is similar immunologically to plasma very-low-density lipoprotein (VLDL) and low-density lipoprotein (LDL) but chemically and physically shows some uniqueness. It has been suggested that VLDL in plasma may represent chylomicrons of varying densities. The role of apolipoproteins in fat absorption and metabolism remains an area of active investigation.

Abnormalities in Lipid Assimilation

Impaired lipid assimilation is considered under the general title of malabsorption. In most cases, all nutrients are malabsorbed to some extent. However, the clinical entity is defined in terms of fat malabsorption because, unlike carbohydrates and proteins, fat not absorbed in the small intestine passes through the colon and appears in the feces in a measurable form.

The presence of excessive fat in the stool, **steatorrhea**, can be established by extracting fecal samples with organic solvents and determining the total fatty acids present, excluding volatile short-chain acids. Less than 7 g of fecal fatty acid per day is normal. Values greater than this level suggest malabsorption or the carcinoid syndrome.

A convenient way to consider fat malabsorption is to review the various steps in assimilation and consider possible derangements in each. For each derangement, at least one possible disease has been recognized:

- Disorders of gastric mixing and intestinal motility do not have any clear-cut disease association, although malabsorption may follow the rapid gastric emptying that accompanies partial gastrectomy. In addition, rapid intestinal transit has been suggested as the basis for diarrhea in hyperthyroidism.

- Luminal digestion of triglycerides may be deranged by defects in pancreatic enzyme secretion or action. A quantitative defect would be caused by impaired enzyme synthesis and secretion, as occurs with cystic fibrosis (a congenital disease of exocrine glands) or chronic pancreatitis. Normal digestion can proceed with as little as 5% to 10% of normal enzyme secretion. A qualitative defect would occur if the conditions for enzyme action were not optimal (as in gastric acid hypersecretion [Zollinger-Ellison syndrome], when the pH of the duodenal contents is lowered and lipase cannot function or may even be denatured). A defect in pancreatic lipase results in the presence of triglycerides in the stool.

- Transport from the lumen is a special step in fat absorption and depends on a suitable bile acid concentration, which may be low because of a quantitative bile acid deficiency that occurs with an interrupted **enterohepatic circulation** (e.g., ileal resection or dysfunction, biliary obstruction, or cholestatic liver disease). There may be a qualitative deficit of the bile acids in a condition known as the *bacterial overgrowth syndrome* (in which stasis in the upper intestine leads to bacterial overgrowth, with deconjugation of bile acids by the bacteria). Free bile acids are absorbed passively in the jejunum because they are largely unionized at the duodenal pH. Bile acids need to be ionized to form micelles. Therefore, the un-ionized state leads to impairment of fat absorption as well as impaired absorption of cholesterol and fat-soluble vitamins. Bile acid deficiency does not interfere with digestion, so in this case free fatty acids and monoglycerides appear in the stool.

- Mucosal cell transport is, of course, necessary for all nutrients, but it is of particular importance in fat absorption because the absorbed fatty acids or monoglycerides must be reconstituted to triglycerides and then formed into chylomicrons. No disease has been associated with triglyceride synthesis; however, there is a disease of inadequate chylomicron formation called *abetalipoprotein-emia*. This condition is caused by a failure to synthesize MTP, which is necessary for the initial steps that bring apolipoprotein B together with triglyceride in the process of chylomicron formation. The synthesis of apolipoprotein B is in fact normal in affected persons, so the condition is misnamed.

- Lymphatic transport is necessary for the absorption of fat that has been reconstituted to chylomicrons. This step is defective in two rare diseases, congenital lymphangiectasia and Whipple's disease.

Thus, by considering the steps in fat absorption, it is possible to predict the diseases that can lead to malabsorption. Steatorrhea, which attends malabsorption, can be alleviated to a large degree by diets containing triglycerides of medium- rather than long-chain fatty acids. The explanation for the benefit of this dietary maneuver is that glycerol esters of medium-chain fatty acids are hydrolyzed faster than are ester linkages involving long-chain fatty acids. Medium-chain fatty acids are water soluble and can be absorbed from aqueous solution. In addition, they are transported directly into portal blood without involvement of chylomicrons.

VITAMINS

Vitamins are organic compounds that cannot be manufactured by the body but are vital for metabolism. They are considered (in this instance) not on the basis of any physiologic function, but rather on the basis of whether they are water soluble or fat soluble (Table 11-3). This feature is emphasized because their solubility dictates the general mechanism by which vitamins are absorbed.

Water-soluble vitamins are represented by an array of compounds. The principles that apply to the absorption of hexoses and amino acids apply to the absorption of vitamins as well. Strongly ionized or high-molecular-weight compounds are absorbed poorly compared with nonionized, low-molecular-weight substances.

Relatively little information exists regarding the processes involved in the intestinal uptake of vitamins.

TABLE 11-3 Solubility of Vitamins		
Vitamin	**Fat Soluble**	**Water Soluble**
A	+	
B_1 (thiamine)		+
B_2 (riboflavin)		+
Niacin		+
C (ascorbic acid)		+
D	+	
E	+	
K	+	
Folic acid		+
B_6 (pyridoxine, pyridoxal, pyridoxamine)		+
B_{12}		+
Pantothenic acid		+
Biotin		+

Most evidence suggests that passive diffusion is the predominant mechanism. Exceptions exist for thiamine, vitamin C, folic acid, and vitamin B_{12}, for which special transport mechanisms have been reported.

At low luminal concentrations, thiamine (vitamin B_1) can be absorbed in the jejunum of some species, including humans, by an Na^+-dependent, active process, whereas at high concentrations, passive diffusion predominates. The presence of a carrier-mediated transport system is suggested by the finding that metabolic inhibitors, thiamine analogues, and the absence of Na^+ all depress thiamine uptake by enterocytes. Riboflavin (vitamin B_2) is absorbed in the proximal small bowel by facilitated transport. Pyridoxine (vitamin B_6) is absorbed by simple diffusion.

Vitamin C is required in only a few species, including humans. Humans are capable of absorbing it from the intestine by passive processes and also by active transport (an energy-dependent process, requiring Na^+). In rats and hamsters, species that do not require ascorbic acid, uptake of the vitamin occurs only by passive mechanisms.

Folic acid has been reported as being transported actively in the duodenum and jejunum of humans and from the entire small intestine of some rodents. A mediated process may be predicted from two facts: folic acid is a strongly electronegative compound (with a molecular weight of 441), and uncouplers of respiration (hence energy production) interfere with its absorption.

Vitamin B_{12} (cobalamin) absorption requires intrinsic factor, a glycoprotein secreted by the parietal cell of the gastric mucosa. Binding of intrinsic factor to dietary vitamin B_{12} is necessary for attachment to specific receptors located in the brush border of the ileum. Initially cobalamin is released from foods by food preparation and exposure to light. It is then recognized by the cobalamin binding protein, haptocorrin (a glycoprotein), which in humans is secreted in saliva and is resistant to digestion by acid and pepsin. Thus haptocorrin protects intrinsic factor during its transit through the stomach. In the duodenum, the haptocorrin is digested by pancreatic enzymes, and the vitamin then forms a complex with intrinsic factor that is resistant to digestion. The presence of calcium (Ca^{2+}) or magnesium (Mg^{2+}) and an alkaline pH are necessary for optimal attachment of the intrinsic factor–B_{12} complex to the receptor, a process that does not require energy. The actual uptake of B_{12} is presumed to be by pinocytosis; however, this point is not clear. Any disease condition that interferes with the production or secretion of intrinsic factor or with the attachment of the intrinsic factor–B_{12} complex to its receptor in the ileum leads to malabsorption of vitamin B_{12}.

The fat-soluble vitamins (A, D, E, and K) depend on solubilization within bile salt micelles for intestinal absorption. Vitamin A, or retinol, is ingested as β-carotene and absorbed as such. Once in the enterocyte, β-carotene is cleaved intracellularly into two retinol molecules. Esters of dietary vitamins D and E, as noted earlier in this chapter, are digested by cholesterol ester hydrolase before their solubilization in micelles. Dietary vitamin K (K_1) is absorbed in the intestine by an active transport system, whereas bacterially derived K_2 is taken up passively from the lumen. Except for retinol, which is reesterified, the fat-soluble vitamins appear in exocytosed chylomicrons biochemically unaltered by metabolic processes within the enterocyte. The chylomicrons are then extruded into the lymphatics and transported via the thoracic duct into the blood. Thus the absorption of fat-soluble vitamins depends on the absorption of dietary lipids. In fact, a fatty meal is necessary for absorption of reasonable amounts of vitamin E. Defects leading to fat malabsorption result in deficiencies of fat-soluble vitamins.

Abnormality in Vitamin Absorption

Pernicious anemia occurs when the body does not make enough red blood cells because of malabsorption of vitamin B_{12}. The most common cause is the failure to secrete sufficient intrinsic factor, which is usually the result of atrophic gastritis and the absence of parietal cells. This is an autoimmune condition, and the body produces parietal cell antibodies that destroy the intrinsic factor–secreting parietal cells. In rare instances pernicious anemia can be caused by the absence of pancreatic proteases and the failure of intrinsic factor to be released from haptocorrin so that it cannot bind vitamin B_{12}. Surgical removal of the ileum also results in pernicious anemia because that is the only site of vitamin B_{12} absorption. The liver stores a 3- to 5-year supply of vitamin B_{12}, so patients do not show symptoms of the condition until several years after it develops. The condition is treated by vitamin B_{12} injections.

SUMMARY

1. Digestion is the chemical breakdown of food by enzymes secreted into the lumen of the gut and those associated with the brush border of enterocytes.
2. All physiologically significant absorption of nutrients occurs in the small intestine, the mucosal surface of which is greatly increased, thus providing a large area for uptake.
3. The major luminal breakdown of carbohydrates is catalyzed by amylase. Breakdown of remaining glucose polymers and other disaccharides is carried out by specific enzymes in the brush border membrane. Glucose and galactose share an Na^+-dependent, secondary active transport mechanism for absorption.
4. The major enzymes involved in the luminal digestion of protein are secreted in inactive forms by the pancreas and are then activated by trypsin following its own activation by enterokinase.
5. Dipeptides, tripeptides, and amino acids are absorbed across the brush border membrane by a variety of transport processes. Larger peptides are

broken down into these absorbable forms by peptidases associated with the brush border. Absorbed small peptides are hydrolyzed to amino acids within the cytoplasm, and almost all absorbed protein leaves the enterocyte in the form of amino acids.

6. Fat droplets are suspended in an emulsification by the action of lecithin, bile salts, peptides, and other such agents. Colipase displaces a bile salt molecule from the fat-water interface, thereby allowing pancreatic lipase to digest the triglycerides. Pancreatic lipase is essential to fat digestion and produces 2-monoglycerides and free fatty acids.

7. The breakdown products of fat digestion are solubilized in micelles by bile salts and other amphipathic molecules. Micelles diffuse through the unstirred layer, and fat digestion products are absorbed from the micelles at the enterocyte brush border membrane.

8. Within the enterocyte, triglycerides and phospholipids are resynthesized and packaged into chylomicrons that contain apoprotein on their surface. Chylomicrons are exocytosed into the intercellular space. Too large to enter capillaries, the chylomicrons enter lacteals and eventually reach the blood via the thoracic lymph duct.

K E Y   W O R D S   A N D   C O N C E P T S

Brush border	Facilitated diffusion
Enterocytes	Active transport
Goblet cells	Starch
Paneth cells	Steatorrhea
Digestion	Sucrose
Luminal/cavital digestion	Lactose
Contact/membrane digestion	Maltose
Unstirred layer of fluid	Amylopectin
Glycocalyx	Lactase deficiency
Passive diffusion	Endopeptidases
	Exopeptidases

Trypsinogen	Colipase
Enterokinase	Phospholipase A_2
Chymotrypsinogen	Cholesterol esterase
Proelastase	Nonspecific esterase
Procarboxypeptidases A and B	Micelles
Triglycerides	Critical micellar concentration
Phospholipids	Enterohepatic circulation
Sterols	Fatty acid–binding proteins
Emulsification	Chylomicrons
Carboxyl ester lipase	Apolipoprotein
Gastric lipase	
Pancreatic lipase	

SUGGESTED READINGS

Ahnen DJ: Nutrient assimilation. In Kelly WN, editor: *Textbook of Internal Medicine*, Philadelphia, 1989, Lippincott.

Ganapathy V: Protein digestion and absorption. In Johnson LR, editor: ed 5, *Physiology of the Gastrointestinal Tract*, vol 2, San Diego, 2012, Elsevier.

Hamilton RL, Wong JS, Cham CM, et al: Chylomicron-sized lipid particles are formed in the setting of apolipoprotein B deficiency, *J Lipid Res* 39:1543–1557, 1998.

Mansbach CM II, Abumrad NA: Enterocyte fatty acid handling proteins and chylomicron formation. In Johnson LR, editor: ed 5, *Physiology of the Gastrointestinal Tract*, vol 2, San Diego, 2012, Elsevier.

Milne MD: Hereditary disorders of intestinal transport. In Smythe DH, editor: *Intestinal Absorption*, New York, 1974, Plenum Press.

Said HM, Nexo E: Mechanism and regulation of intestinal absorption of water-soluble vitamins: cellular and molecular aspects. In Johnson LR, editor: ed 5, *Physiology of the Gastrointestinal Tract*, vol 2, San Diego, 2012, Elsevier.

Tso P: Intestinal lipid absorption. In Johnson LR, editor: *Physiology of the Gastrointestinal Tract*, ed 3, New York, 1994, Raven Press.

Wellner D, Meister A: A survey of inborn errors of amino acid metabolism and transport in man, *Annu Rev Biochem* 50: 911–968, 1980.

Whitcomb DC: Hereditary pancreatitis: new insights into acute and chronic pancreatitis, *Gut* 45:317–322, 1999.

Wright EM, Sal-Rabanal M, Loo DDF, Hirayama BA: Sugar absorption. In Johnson LR, editor: ed 5, *Physiology of the Gastrointestinal Tract*, vol 2, San Diego, 2012, Elsevier.

12 FLUID AND ELECTROLYTE ABSORPTION

OBJECTIVES

- Indicate the sources of fluid and electrolytes in the GI tract and their sites of absorption.
- Describe the mechanisms involved in and the location of the sites for the absorption of sodium, potassium, chloride, bicarbonate, and water.
- Understand the mechanism and significance of the intestinal secretion of fluid and electrolytes.
- Explain the difference between osmotic and secretory diarrheas and discuss the disorders that may lead to each.
- Discuss the basic steps involved in the absorption of calcium and iron and how each is regulated.

Minerals and water enter the body through the intestine and provide the solutes and solvent water for body fluids. The electrolytes of primary importance include sodium (Na^+), potassium (K^+), hydrogen ion (H^+), bicarbonate (HCO_3^-), chloride (Cl^-), calcium (Ca^{2+}), and iron (Fe^{2+}). Each of these ions has one or more mechanisms by which it is transported across the intestinal epithelium. This chapter considers these mechanisms and their relationship with water absorption and secretion.

BIDIRECTIONAL FLUID FLUX

During a 24-hour period, 7 to 10 L of water enters the small intestine (Fig. 12-1). Fluid derived from food and drink accounts for approximately 2 L. The other 7 L is derived from the secretions of the gastrointestinal (GI) tract: saliva, 1 L; gastric juice, 2 L; pancreatic juice, 2 L; bile, 1 L; and small intestinal secretions, 1 L. Of the amount entering, only approximately 600 mL per 24-hour period reaches the colon, a finding indicating that most water is absorbed in the small intestine. Because the average daily fecal weight is approximately 150 g, of which 100 g is water, 500 mL of fluid is absorbed daily from the colon. This volume represents 10% to 25% of the absorptive capacity of the colon, which can absorb approximately 4 to 6 L of fluid per day. Malabsorption of solutes and water in the small intestine may permit enough fluid to enter the colon to overwhelm its absorptive capacity and cause diarrhea. This, in turn, can precipitate severe electrolyte deficiencies. Although it is possible that ions and water may be added to the feces from colonic mucosa, the major source of water and electrolytes in a diarrheic stool is the small intestine (see Fig. 12-1).

It is evident from the foregoing account that several liters of fluid are secreted into the GI tract daily, and several liters are absorbed. The volume of fluid moving from blood to lumen (secretion) is less than that moving from the lumen to the blood (absorption), thus resulting in net absorption. Absorption generally results from the passive movement of water across the epithelial membrane in response to osmotic and hydrostatic pressures. Because of these so-called *Starling forces,* the consequent bulk flow of fluid is analogous to the flow of fluid across capillary walls. In the absence of food, ions are the most important contributors to osmotic pressure in the intestinal lumen. The ionic composition of the luminal contents may vary along the length of the intestine and is different from that in feces. Luminal fluid generally remains isotonic

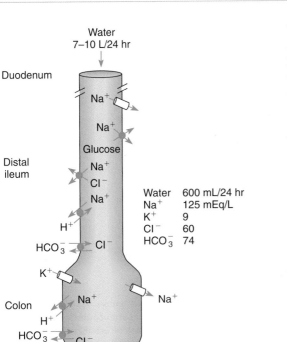

FIGURE 12-1 ■ Volume and composition of fluid entering and leaving the gastrointestinal tract during 24 hours. The locations of the various ion transporters are shown along with the volume and composition of the fluid leaving the small intestine and the colon. Cl^-, chloride; H^+, hydrogen ion; HCO_3^-, bicarbonate; K^+, potassium; Na^+, sodium.

with plasma, however, because of the relative permeability of the mucosal membrane. The continued production of solutes by colonic bacteria, together with the relative impermeability of the colonic membrane to water, usually causes stool water to be hypertonic, 350 to 400 milliosmoles (mOsm)/L, to plasma.

IONIC CONTENT OF LUMINAL FLUID

Osmotic equilibration with plasma of material entering the small bowel occurs rapidly in the duodenum.

Water is absorbed from hypotonic solutions and enters hypertonic solutions. Na^+ and Cl^- also leave hypertonic solutions. Most of this movement occurs through the relatively permeable junctions between the epithelial cells of the proximal small intestine.

Proceeding from the duodenum to the colon, the Na^+ and Cl^- concentrations in the lumen progressively become lower than the plasma concentrations. In the duodenum, the concentration of Na^+ is approximately 140 mEq/L, equal to the serum concentration. The major anion is Cl^-. Na^+ concentrations decrease in the jejunum and reach approximately 125 mEq/L in the ileum. The major anions in the ileum are Cl^- and HCO_3^-. Na^+ decreases to 35 to 40 mEq/L in the colon, whereas the K^+ concentration increases to 90 mEq/L, up from 9 mEq/L in the ileum. The major anions in the colon are Cl^- and HCO_3^-.

These values indicate an effective absorption process for Na^+ that becomes increasingly efficient toward the distal portions of the gut. This is caused in part by a decrease in the permeability of the epithelium that prevents the back-diffusion of ions absorbed in the distal portions. Whereas the absorption of Na^+ in the distal gut is effective, the conservation of Cl^- is even more so. Cl^- is exchanged for metabolically derived HCO_3^-.

K^+ is absorbed passively by the small intestine as the volume of intestinal contents decreases. The concentration of K^+ remains roughly equal to that in the serum (4 or 5 mEq/L). In the colon, net K^+ secretion occurs. Because of K^+ secretion and the exchange of Cl^- for HCO_3^- in the colon, prolonged diarrhea results in hypokalemic metabolic acidosis.

TRANSPORT ROUTES AND PROCESSES

Ions move between the gut lumen and the blood through **transcellular** and **paracellular pathways.** The passive movement of Na^+, both into and out of the lumen, is largely through the lateral spaces. This movement is determined by the **tight junctions** or **zonulae occludens.** The rate of this passive component is affected by electrochemical gradients and Starling forces. Normally these forces are small and account for only a small fraction of the net transport. They can, however, be altered under certain conditions, with marked effects.

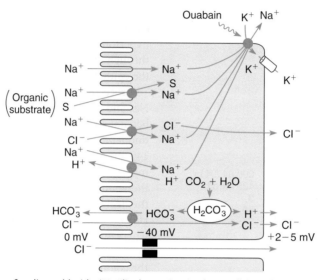

FIGURE 12-2 ■ Mechanism of sodium chloride (NaCl) absorption in the small intestine. Na$^+$ enters passively, following the electrochemical gradient, by cotransport with nutrients such as glucose or amino acids, or by neutral cotransport with Cl$^-$ or in exchange for protons via a countertransport process. Cl$^-$ also is absorbed by neutral exchange with bicarbonate (HCO$_3^-$). Na$^+$ exit from the cell is via the energy-dependent Na$^+$ pump, and Cl$^-$ follows passively. The electrical potential difference across the apical membrane is –40 mV, and across the entire cell is +2 to +5 mV with reference to the luminal side. Ouabain is an inhibitor of Na$^+$, potassium (K$^+$)-adenosine triphosphatase (ATPase). H$^+$, hydrogen ion; H$_2$CO$_3^-$, carbonic acid.

The tight junction is about twice as permeable to Na$^+$ and K$^+$ as it is to Cl$^-$. Thus electrical potentials can arise across this structure. If, for example, NaCl is moving across the tight junction, the Cl$^-$ will be retarded relative to the Na$^+$, and the surface toward which the movement is occurring will become positive relative to the other surface. Ions slightly larger than Na$^+$ and K$^+$ are much more restricted in their movement.

The pores through which transcellular diffusion takes place are probably larger (7 to 8 angstroms [Å]) in the proximal bowel than in the ileum (3 to 4 Å). This restricts the passive transport of solutes in the distal gut and allows these solutes to exert a more effective osmotic pressure. In turn, the reduced permeability makes carrier-mediated transport a more important contributor to net transport out of the lumen.

Sodium-Chloride Transport

Physiologic models describing Na$^+$ and Cl$^-$ absorption in the small intestine are shown in Figure 12-2. Na$^+$ is absorbed from the lumen across the apical membrane of epithelial cells by four mechanisms. These include the movement of Na$^+$ by restricted diffusion through water-filled channels, the cotransport of Na$^+$ with organic solutes (e.g., glucose and amino acids), the cotransport of Na$^+$ with Cl$^-$, and the countertransport of Na$^+$ in exchange for H$^+$. Because Na$^+$-Cl$^-$ cotransport and Na$^+$-H$^+$ exchange are electrically neutral processes, the driving force for Na$^+$ to enter the cell is the Na$^+$ concentration difference between the luminal fluid and the cytoplasm. Na$^+$ movement through pores and Na$^+$ cotransport with organic solutes are also driven by the Na$^+$ concentration difference but are electrogenic and increase the negative electrical potential across the epithelial cell membrane. The contribution of restricted diffusion to overall Na$^+$ absorption is probably small relative to other mechanisms.

The presence of these various mechanisms varies over the length of the small intestine. In the proximal bowel, Na$^+$ is absorbed primarily coupled to H$^+$ countertransport and solute (amino acids and sugars) cotransport. In the ileum, Na$^+$ is absorbed coupled to the absorption of Cl$^-$. Throughout the gut, Cl$^-$ is absorbed along the electrical gradient. In the ileum, coupled Na$^+$ transport is the major carrier-mediated pathway for Cl$^-$ absorption. Exchange of Cl$^-$ for HCO$_3^-$

occurs in the distal ileum and increases dramatically in the colon and rectum. This mechanism accounts for the high HCO_3^- content and alkaline pH of stool water.

The Na^+-K^+ pump on the basolateral membranes of the absorbing epithelial cell maintains both the low intracellular Na^+ level and the negative membrane potential. The Na^+ that enters by all four mechanisms described previously is extruded into the intercellular spaces by the Na^+ pump, which is the well-known Na^+,K^+-activated adenosine triphosphatase (ATPase). This enzyme-carrier molecule is activated by intracellular Na^+ and extracellular K^+ to split adenosine triphosphate (ATP), thereby releasing energy. In the process, three Na^+ ions are pumped out of the cell for every two K^+ ions pumped into it. The pumping out of more Na^+ than there is K^+ entering creates a potential difference (PD) across the basolateral membrane, which is called an **electrogenic potential.** The pump is inhibited by cardiac glycosides (e.g., ouabain). Because Na^+ exit from the epithelial cell is coupled with K^+ entry, the intracellular K^+ concentration is much higher than the extracellular concentration. This causes the constant, downhill leakage of K^+ from the interior to the exterior by K^+ channels on the basolateral membranes (i.e., the K^+ actively pumped into the cell returns to the exterior through passive leaks).

The epithelial absorption of Cl^- involves, in addition to cotransport with Na^+, countertransport with HCO_3^- (see Fig. 12-2). HCO_3^- is produced by a metabolic process within the epithelial cells through the hydration of carbon dioxide (CO_2) by carbonic anhydrase. Both absorptive mechanisms move Cl^- into the epithelial cell against an electrochemical PD. The energy for the uphill movement of Cl^- is derived from the downhill movement of Na^+ into the cell or from the downhill movement of HCO_3^- out of the cell and into the lumen.

Because of the transcellular electrical PD (the serosal side is positive with reference to the lumen and with reference to the cell interior), Cl^- is driven passively from the cell and into the serosal fluid. In addition, luminal Cl^- can move through the paracellular pathway into the serosal solution. The magnitude of this passive absorptive process is governed by the magnitude of the transmural PD. That PD is developed through the action of the Na^+-K^+ pump and the absorption of Na^+ coupled to organic solutes. It is influenced by the resistance of the paracellular pathway to ion flow. In the small intestine, the relatively leaky epithelium prevents the transmural PD from rising to more than 2 to 5 millivolts (mV). In the colon, where the epithelium is less leaky, the PD is approximately 20 mV. Thus the driving force for Cl^- absorption is greater in the colon.

All regions of the colon absorb Na^+ and Cl^- (Fig. 12-3). Unlike in the small intestine, however, the cotransport of Na^+ with organic solutes is lacking. Restricted diffusion is the primary mechanism for colonic Na^+ absorption. This electrogenic process, which increases in activity from oral to aboral regions, depends on channels that are under regulation by mineralocorticoids. For example, aldosterone increases the number of Na^+ channels and enhances Na^+ absorption. Na^+ in the lumen of the colon also is absorbed through an electroneutral process that includes Cl^- cotransport. This probably involves Na^+-H^+ countertransport coupled with Cl^--HCO_3^- countertransport, as occurs in the small intestine. This secretion of HCO_3^- accounts for the alkalinity of stool water.

Potassium Transport

Diffusion through paracellular pathways in the small intestine is the primary mechanism by which K^+, derived from the diet or from secretions of the upper GI tract, undergoes net absorption. In the colon (but not in the small intestine), the apical and basolateral membranes are permeable to K^+. Thus because of the high concentration of intracellular K^+ maintained by the Na^+-K^+ pump, some K^+ leaks passively across the apical membrane of epithelial cells. Factors that elevate intracellular K^+, such as aldosterone-stimulated Na^+ absorption, increase K^+ secretion. Therefore, aldosterone conserves body Na^+ at the expense of K^+.

MECHANISM FOR WATER ABSORPTION AND SECRETION

Water absorption or secretion always occurs in response to osmotic forces produced by the transport of organic solutes or ions and can be explained in terms of a three-compartment model and local osmotic effects (Fig. 12-4). In the absorbing intestine, solutes are moved from the lumen (first compartment) into and then out of the epithelial cell. This creates a local osmotic gradient that causes water to move from the

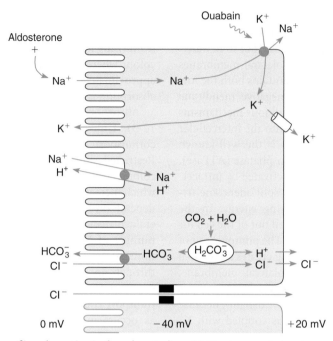

FIGURE 12-3 ■ Mechanism of ion absorption in the colon. Sodium (Na^+) enters passively, whereas chloride (Cl^-) enters in neutral exchange with bicarbonate (HCO_3^-). Net secretion of potassium (K^+) occurs. H^+, hydrogen ion.

gut lumen, across the cell, and into the intercellular space (second compartment). The entrance of water increases the hydrostatic pressure within this space and causes the bulk flow of water and solutes through the basement membrane into capillaries (third compartment). In the nonabsorbing intestine, the imbalance of forces across the capillary wall leads to filtration of fluid into the interstitium. However, the capillary filtration rate is balanced by lymphatic drainage. In the secreting intestine, fluid in the interstitium is attracted osmotically into the lumen.

Osmotic equilibration and thus absorption occur by different means in the duodenum and the ileum. The duodenum functions to bring chyme into osmotic equilibrium with plasma. If a hypertonic solution is placed in the duodenum, isotonicity is reached by a rapid flow of water from blood to lumen, thereby increasing the volume of the original solution. More distally, in the small intestine, absorption of solutes creates a gradient for water absorption. Thus the volume is decreased because of both solute and water uptake, and the isotonicity of the luminal solution is maintained during this process. In summary, the sequence of responses to hypertonic contents entering the intestinal lumen is the following: (1) the dilution caused by osmotic attraction of water from the blood and (2) the movement of fluid from the lumen into the blood secondary to the transport of solutes.

If a hypotonic solution enters the intestine, the flux of water from lumen to blood is greater than from blood to lumen and leads to net absorption of fluid. This in turn is followed by the isotonic uptake of fluid.

The gut normally absorbs all electrolytes and water presented to it and, unlike the kidney, does not appear subject to hour-by-hour homeostatic regulation. Nevertheless, some external regulation occurs. The autonomic nervous system has effects on NaCl transport. Adrenergic (α-receptor) or anticholinergic stimuli tend to increase absorption, but cholinergic or antiadrenergic stimuli tend to decrease absorption. Other agents (e.g., serotonin, dopamine, the endogenous opiates, enkephalins, and endorphins) alter gut transport, usually in the secretory direction. However, the opiates morphine and codeine increase gut absorption.

The ileum has relatively little ability to respond to Na^+ depletion and/or mineralocorticoids. By contrast,

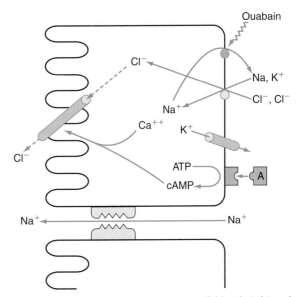

FIGURE 12-5 ■ Model for the secretion of chloride (Cl⁻) and sodium (Na⁺) by the crypt cells of the small and large intestines. A, agonist; ATP, adenosine triphosphate; cAMP, cyclic adenosine monophosphate; K⁺, potassium.

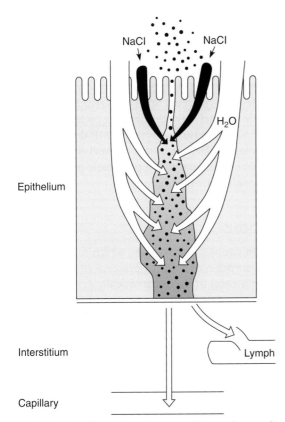

FIGURE 12-4 ■ Fluid absorption according to the standing osmotic gradient hypothesis. The sum of hydrostatic and osmotic pressures in the intraepithelial space, interstitium, and capillaries favors fluid absorption. In the nonabsorbing state, fluid filtering from the capillaries would be drained by the lymphatics. The attraction of fluid from the cytosol and interstitium secondary to high osmotic pressure in the lumen leads to secretion. NaCl, sodium chloride.

the large intestine is sensitive to both these assaults, which can increase Na⁺ absorption and K⁺ secretion. Mineralocorticoids can decrease the Na⁺ concentration in fecal water from 30 to 2 mEq/L and increase the K⁺ concentration from 75 to 150 mEq/L. The influence of aldosterone on Na⁺ transport is exerted at two points. There is an increase in Na⁺ permeability of the brush border membrane caused by the activation of new Na⁺ channels. In addition, aldosterone apparently increases the number of Na⁺ pump molecules in the basolateral membrane.

Factors that cause the osmotic retention of water in the gut lumen or stimulate fluid secretion may lead to diarrhea. Saline laxatives such as Epsom salts (magnesium sulfate [$MgSO_4$]) increase fecal water because of the slow and incomplete absorption of polyvalent ions. Disease states such as disaccharidase deficiency or monosaccharide malabsorption increase the amount of unabsorbed solutes entering the colon and cause **osmotic diarrhea.**

INTESTINAL SECRETION

Both the small and the large intestines secrete water and electrolytes. This process resides primarily in the crypt cells and is responsible for maintaining a liquid chyme.

The transcellular secretion of Cl⁻ accounts for most of the secretory activity, and the mechanism is illustrated in Figure 12-5. Cl⁻ enters the cell through a carrier located in the basolateral membrane. The carrier uses the Na⁺ gradient established by the Na⁺,K⁺-ATPase to move Cl⁻ into the cell against its electrochemical gradient. Two Cl⁻ are moved into the cell along with one Na⁺ and one K⁺ via this NaK2Cl cotransporter. The Na⁺ entering the cell is extruded by the Na⁺ pump, and K⁺ diffuses back out of the cell through channels in the basolateral membrane. Cl^- enters the lumen through channels in the apical membrane, and Na^+ moves through paracellular pathways, driven by the lumen-negative PD created by the secretion of Cl^-. The resulting secretion of Na^+ and Cl^- establishes an osmotic gradient that draws water into the lumen.

The apical membranes of the crypt cells contain at least two different Cl^- channels. One is activated by increases in intracellular Ca^{2+} and is stimulated by acetylcholine released by the enteric nervous system. The other type is stimulated by agents that increase cyclic adenosine monophosphate (cAMP) and is identical to the cystic fibrosis transmembrane conductance regulator (CFTR) that also is found in pancreatic and airway epithelial cells. Agents such as vasoactive intestinal peptide (VIP), secretin, and prostaglandin that stimulate this channel activate adenylate cyclase to increase cAMP, which in turn activates cAMP-dependent protein kinase A. Defects in this channel account for the intestinal, pulmonary, and pancreatic problems associated with cystic fibrosis.

CLINICAL APPLICATIONS

Diarrhea is a major cause of death or disability in the world today, and it affects individuals of all ages. Death is the direct or indirect result of hypovolemia and circulatory collapse compounded by metabolic acidosis and hypokalemia.

Secretion that is stimulated by gastrointestinal hormones and neurotransmitters after a meal is a physiologic aid to digestion and serves to maintain a liquid chyme during the process of absorption. However, excessive chloride (Cl^-) secretion, with accompanying fluid secretion, can become pathologic. The resulting **secretory diarrheas** are prevalent in many developing nations and constitute a leading cause of death. In some instances this disorder can result from excessive blood levels of normal secretagogues such as vasoactive intestinal peptide, which can be produced by certain tumors. In most cases, however, secretory diarrhea is caused by infection of the gut by pathogenic bacteria such as *Vibrio cholerae* and *Escherichia coli*. These bacteria produce enterotoxins that bind to receptors on the apical membranes of crypt cells. Receptor binding permanently activates the adenylate cyclase located on the basolateral membrane, and the cell is stimulated to secrete maximally for its lifetime. Huge volumes of water and electrolytes may be secreted, so that the absorptive capacity of the gut is greatly exceeded. Unless proper therapy is available, dehydration and death can result.

The presence of sugars or amino acids in the lumen leads to their absorption by the sodium-coupled mechanism, which also leads to the absorption of a Cl^- to preserve electrical neutrality, a total of three osmotically active solutes. This finding led to the suggestion that orally administered saline solutions containing glucose and amino acids could reduce salt and water loss from secretory diarrheas. These oral replacement or rehydration therapies have markedly reduced death and disabilities worldwide and especially in areas where cholera is a problem.

The second and more common type of diarrhea is **osmotic diarrhea**, which can have a variety of causes, each of which leads to the accumulation within the small intestine of nonabsorbable solutes. As discussed earlier, because the small intestine is leaky to water, the luminal contents are always isotonic to plasma. It follows then that the accumulation of nonabsorbable, osmotically active solutes will generate an osmotic difference that draws fluid into the lumen. The absence of certain enzymes such as lactase, for example, results in the accumulation of their substrates. Inadequate bile salt secretion or the inactivation of pancreatic lipase can cause steatorrhea, which is accompanied by water loss. Increased rate of transit of material through the small bowel may not provide sufficient time for absorption. In this case the solutes are absorbable, but they are not in contact with the absorbing surface long enough. Decreases in the amount of the absorbing surface can also cause diarrhea as in cases of infection, inflammation, or allergies, such as gluten-sensitive enteropathy.

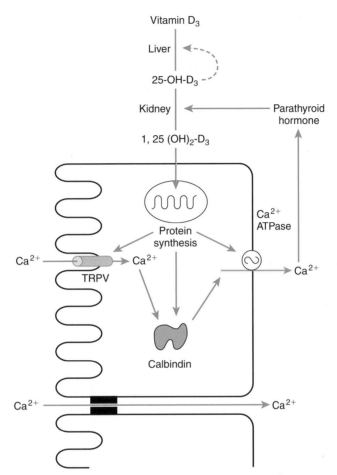

FIGURE 12-6 ▓ Calcium (Ca^{2+}) absorption by an enterocyte within a larger scheme of Ca^{2+} homeostasis. Vitamin D_3, 1,25-$(OH)_2$-D_3, stimulates Ca^{2+} transport by interacting with nuclear receptors to control the synthesis of a Ca^{2+} channel (TRPV6), a calcium-binding protein (calbindin), and the Ca adenosine triphosphatase (ATPase). During periods of high intake, Ca^{2+} is also absorbed paracellularly.

CALCIUM ABSORPTION

Absorption of Ca^{2+} by enterocytes is an important component in the regulation of whole-body Ca^{2+} (Fig. 12-6). The transepithelial movement of the cation occurs against an electrochemical potential. The process, although not entirely known, is localized in the proximal small intestine. Ca^{2+} transport occurs in three major steps. First, Ca^{2+} absorption involves entry at the brush border membrane. Second, a mechanism must be present to regulate intracellular Ca^{2+} levels to prevent altered cell function. Third, Ca^{2+} exit occurs at the basolateral membrane. The synthesis of the

proteins involved in each of these steps is regulated by **vitamin D**.

Transport of Ca^{2+} is initiated by 1,25-dihydroxyvitamin D_3 (1,25-$[OH]_2$-D_3). This active product is derived from vitamin D_3 (cholecalciferol) formed in the skin by the action of ultraviolet radiation on 7-dehydrocholesterol. Vitamin D_3 is transferred to the liver and converted to 25-OH-D_3. The kidney, through a step regulated by parathyroid hormone, converts 25-OH-D_3 to 1,25-$(OH)_2$-D_3. Enterocytes take up the 1,25-$(OH)_2$-D_3, where it reacts with a receptor molecule in the nucleus. The transcription of specific deoxyribonucleic acid (DNA) and protein synthesis are mandatory steps in the action of 1,25-$(OH)_2$-D_3 on Ca^{2+} transport. The Ca^{2+}-binding activity of the synthesized proteins correlates with Ca^{2+} transport. Presumably at least one Ca^{2+} channel of the transient receptor potential vanilloid (TRPV) family is inserted into the brush border and facilitates (gates) the entry of Ca^{2+} down an electrochemical gradient.

Once inside the cell, Ca^{2+} interacts with a binding protein, calbindin, to minimize the rise in intracellular free Ca^{2+}. It has been proposed, but not substantiated, that the mitochondria participate in this "buffering" action. The synthesis of this binding protein is a 1,25-$(OH)_2$-D_3–dependent process. Exit of Ca^{2+} at the basolateral membrane is against an electrochemical gradient and occurs via the Ca^{2+}-ATPase, the synthesis of which is also 1,25-$(OH)_2$-D_3–dependent.

Ca^{2+} absorption is regulated over the long term by plasma Ca^{2+} levels. As intestinal absorption of Ca^{2+} rises, plasma Ca^{2+} increases; this change inhibits the secretion of parathyroid hormone. In turn, formation of 1,25-$(OH)_2$-D_3 in the kidney is inhibited (see Fig. 12-6). A reduction in 1,25-$(OH)_2$-D_3 eventually causes Ca^{2+} absorption to wane because the synthesis of new Ca-binding protein will cease. At high intake levels, Ca^{2+} can also be absorbed through the paracellular pathway. Although the mechanism of Ca^{2+} absorption is not a closed issue, the model depicted in Figure 12-6 provides a currently accepted working scheme.

IRON ABSORPTION

Absorption of iron is regulated by total body iron requirements and by the bioavailability of iron. Under physiologic conditions, dietary iron is acquired through transport processes in the proximal small intestine. Although the stomach, ileum, and colon have some capacity for iron absorption, this process is most prevalent in the duodenum and jejunum. Normally, because body iron is conserved, absorption of iron by the gut is low compared with the amount ingested.

Heme (derived from meat) is an important dietary source of iron. After it is absorbed intact by enterocytes, it loses iron from its porphyrin ring. Heme is absorbed by endocytosis and digested by lysosomal enzymes to release free iron. In all other chemical forms, iron is absorbed only to the extent to which it can be released from food in ionizable form. The insoluble complexes of iron with food become more soluble at a low pH. Gastric acid is important in solubilizing iron, and patients with deficient acid secretion absorb less iron. Organic acids such as ascorbic or citric reduce Fe^{3+} to Fe^{2+}, which is absorbed more efficiently. A brush border reductase, duodenal cytochrome b (DCYTB), plays an important role in reducing ferric to ferrous iron. Nonheme iron represents the largest fraction of dietary iron. The cellular mechanism of iron transport has not been completely described. However, a working hypothesis can be synthesized from what is known about the influx of iron across the brush border, its intracellular processing, and its efflux across the basolateral membrane of enterocytes into the circulation (Fig. 12-7).

Once reduced, ferrous iron is transported across the apical surface by divalent metal transporter 1 (DMT1). An inward flux of H^+, dependent on the outward flux of Na^+ established by the Na^+,K^+-ATPase, provides the driving force for the carrier. Within the cell, the fate of the iron depends on the body supply. If body stores are filled, most iron will be stored within **ferritin** and lost when the enterocyte is sloughed into the lumen. If iron stores are low, most will cross the basolateral membrane via the iron export protein ferroprotein 1 (FPN1). During the export process, iron is oxidized for binding to transferrin (TF) in the interstitial fluid and plasma. Oxidation is carried out by the iron oxidase hephaestin (HEPH), which is expressed in the basolateral membrane.

The uptake pathway for heme is not understood in detail, but the HCP1 receptor is probably involved. Heme can be broken down in lysosomes and the iron released for export, or it can exit the cell intact and be bound to hemopexin for distribution to the body.

The body requirement for iron influences intestinal uptake. Absorption is thought to be regulated at a minimum of two sites. First, during iron deficiency, transcription factors are activated that enter the enterocyte nucleus and increase the synthesis the enzyme DCYTB and the iron transporter, DMT1. Second, the amount of the storage protein, ferritin, is also regulated. The formation of ferritin is least when the body iron levels are low. Thus iron transfer out of the duodenal cells to the blood is increased. The reverse holds when iron stores are replete. Intestinal absorption of iron decreases as enzyme and transporter synthesis is decreased, and exit from the enterocytes decreases as the formation of ferritin is increased.

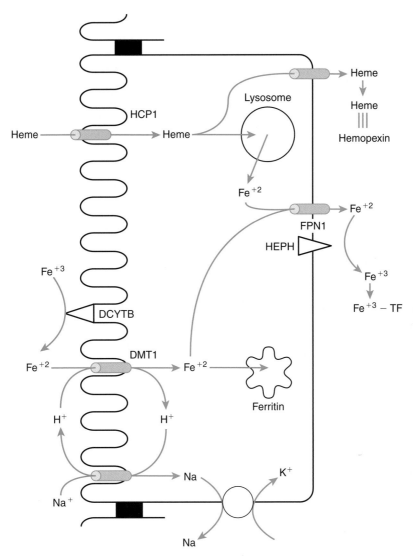

FIGURE 12-7 ■ Inorganic iron (Fe^{3+}) is reduced to the ferrous form (Fe^{2+}) by the reductase, DCYTB, in the apical membrane and is transported into the cell by the divalent metal transporter, DMT1. Some iron is bound to ferritin and stored within the cell. Cytoplasmic iron is pumped out of the cell via ferroprotein 1 (FPN1), oxidized by hephaestin (HEPH), and bound to transferrin (TF) in the interstitial space. H^+, hydrogen ion; K^+, potassium; Na^+, sodium.

SUMMARY

1. Approximately 9 L of water enters the GI tract per day. Of this amount, 2 L is ingested, and 7 L is secreted into the lumen. The small intestine absorbs approximately 8.5 L and the colon 0.4 L, thus leaving only 100 mL to be excreted in the stool.

2. The absorption of water occurs by diffusion down an osmotic gradient created by the absorption of Na^+, Cl^-, other electrolytes, and nutrients such as sugars and amino acids.

3. Four mechanisms account for the absorption of Na^+: passive diffusion, countertransport with H^+, cotransport with organic solutes (sugars and amino acids), and cotransport with Cl^-. The presence of

these mechanisms varies along the length of the bowel.

4. Throughout the bowel, Cl^- is absorbed passively down its electrical gradient. In addition to being absorbed with Na^+, Cl^- is absorbed in the distal ileum and colon in exchange for HCO_3^-, which is secreted into the lumen and accounts for the alkalinity of stool water.

5. Crypt cells contain channels for Cl^- secretion in their apical membranes that respond to increases in cAMP. Various toxins, such as cholera toxin, and GI peptides, such as VIP, trigger secretion via this mechanism, which depends on the Na^+,K^+-ATPase of the basolateral membrane.

6. The small intestine actively absorbs Ca^{2+} by a process dependent on vitamin D, which stimulates the synthesis of a channel protein in the apical membrane, a cytoplasmic binding protein, and Ca ATPase in the basolateral membrane.

7. Most iron is absorbed as inorganic iron. Ferric iron is reduced by the enzyme DCYTB in the brush border to ferrous iron, which is transported into the cell by the divalent metal transporter, DMT1. If body stores are filled, most is bound to ferritin and lost when the cell is shed. During depletion, the iron exits the cell via the FPN1 transporter, is oxidized by HEPH, and is bound to TF and carried in the blood. Heme is also absorbed and can exit the cell intact or be broken down in lysosomes to release ferrous iron.

SUGGESTED READINGS

Binder HJ, Sandle GI: Electrolyte transport in the mammalian colon. In Johnson LR, editor: *Physiology of the Gastrointestinal Tract*, ed 3, New York, 1994, Raven Press.

Chang EB, Rao MC: Intestinal water and electrolyte transport: mechanisms of physiological and adaptive responses. In Johnson LR, editor: *Physiology of the Gastrointestinal Tract*, ed 3, New York, 1994, Raven Press.

Collins JF, Anderson GJ: Molecular mechanisms of intestinal iron transport. In Johnson LR, editor: ed 5, *Physiology of the Gastrointestinal Tract*, vol 2, San Diego, 2012, Elsevier.

Dharmsathaphorn K: Intestinal water and electrolyte transport. In Kelly WN, editor: *Textbook of Internal Medicine*, Philadelphia, 1989, Lippincott.

Kiela PR, Collins JF, Ghishan FK: Molecular mechanisms of intestinal transport of calcium, phosphate, and magnesium. In Johnson LR, editor: ed 5, *Physiology of the Gastrointestinal Tract*, vol 2, San Diego, 2012, Elsevier.

Kiela PR, Ghishan FK: Na^+/H^+ exchange in mammalian digestive tract. In Johnson LR, editor: ed 5, *Physiology of the Gastrointestinal Tract*, vol 2, San Diego, 2012, Elsevier.

Montrose MH: Small intestine, absorption and secretion. In Johnson LR, editor: *Encyclopedia of Gastroenterology*, vol 3, San Diego, 2004, Academic Press, pp 399–404.

Thiagarajah JR, Verkman AS: Water transport in the gastrointestinal tract. In Johnson LR, editor: ed 5, *Physiology of the Gastrointestinal Tract*, vol 2, San Diego, 2012, Elsevier.

KEY WORDS AND CONCEPTS

Transcellular pathways

Paracellular pathways

Tight junctions/zonulae occludens

Electrogenic potential

Osmotic diarrhea

Secretory diarrhea

Vitamin D

Ferritin

REGULATION OF FOOD INTAKE

OBJECTIVES

- Understand the importance of food intake to clinical medicine.
- Discuss the role of the nervous system in the regulation of food intake.
- Explain the role of the endocrine system in the regulation of metabolism and food intake.
- Discuss the role of the gastrointestinal (GI) system in the regulation food intake.
- Understand how input from the nervous, endocrine, and GI systems is integrated to regulate food intake and metabolism.
- Discuss the various treatments for obesity.

The human species evolved during a time when the source of the next meal was highly uncertain. As a result, the gastrointestinal (GI) tract evolved to optimize the processing of ingested material when it became available. Receptive relaxation allows the stomach to accommodate large volumes with minimal increases in gastric pressure. Digestive enzymes are secreted in great excess. The secretion of pancreatic lipase, for example, must be reduced by at least 80% before steatorrhea occurs. There is significant overlap in the specificity of transport proteins or carriers for the absorption of most amino acids. Indeed, even the absorptive surface of the small intestine can be reduced 60% to 70%, as long as sufficient ileum remains to reabsorb bile acids and to absorb vitamin B_{12}, before increased amounts of nutrients appear in the stool.

The result is that virtually all ingested carbohydrate, protein, and fat are broken down and absorbed. It is impossible to saturate the digestive and absorptive capacities of the GI tract. This situation was advantageous when acquiring a meal was uncertain and also required an expenditure of calories in the form of exercise, but now that the nearest meal is available by opening the refrigerator door or, worse, pulling into the parking lot of the nearest convenience store or fast food restaurant, the result is an epidemic of obesity with its sequelae of diabetes, cardiovascular disease, and some forms of cancer.

At present, more than two thirds of Americans are overweight, and one third can be classified as obese. The prevalence of obesity in children has increased markedly. Obesity has now displaced cigarette smoking as the number one health problem in the nation. In the United States approximately 300,000 deaths per year are directly attributed to obesity. In rare cases, obesity can be caused by a gene mutation, but in an overwhelming majority of instances, obesity is the result of a long-term imbalance between intake and expenditure of calories. These two quantities must remain equivalent to maintain body weight. Although a certain amount of weight control can be effected by increasing caloric expenditure in the form of exercise, the fact of the matter is that most of us overeat.

APPETITE CONTROL

In view of the recognized importance of normal body weight for maintaining health, an understanding of the mechanisms regulating food intake seems imperative.

Current knowledge of the regulation of food intake is far from complete, however, and only in the past few years has sufficient evidence been accumulated for inclusion in a textbook of GI physiology. In fact, knowledge about this aspect of the field lags far behind that on the topics covered in other chapters of this book. Another significant difference between this subject and those of the other chapters is that the regulation of food intake depends heavily on contributions from systems other than the digestive system—namely, the endocrine and nervous systems.

THE NERVOUS SYSTEM

Signals affecting food intake are integrated in the brain. These signals include emotions and learned behavior, as well as hormonal and neural input from the endocrine system and the GI tract. Input provides information regarding total energy stores and the presence of nutrients within the digestive tract. In addition, the vagus nerve relays input regarding gastric distention, secretory activity, and the release of various hormones from the stomach and duodenum.

Hypothalamus

Most of the integration of signals affecting food intake takes place in the **arcuate nucleus** of the hypothalamus. Two pathways exist: one inhibiting food intake and increasing metabolism and the other stimulating food intake and inhibiting metabolism (Fig. 13-1). The **melanocortin** pathway is made up of appetite-inhibiting neurons containing pro-opiomelanocortin (POMC), which releases α-melanocyte-stimulating

hormone (α-MSH). α-MSH binds melanocortin receptors (MC4), present on second-order neurons, to inhibit food intake and increase the rate of metabolism. The stimulation of feeding is provided by the **neuropeptide Y** (NPY) pathway. Hunger signals stimulate the release of NPY, which binds to Y1 receptors to increase feeding behavior and the storage of calories. It would make little sense for both these pathways to be operating at the same time, and the NPY system also releases agouti-related peptide (AgRP), which is an antagonist of the MC4 receptor. In addition, peptides that stimulate the melanocortin system inhibit the NPY system. Some cases of obesity in humans have been traced to mutations in the *POMC* and *MC4R* genes. Approximately 5% of cases of childhood obesity have been linked to *MC4R* mutations.

Enteric Nervous System and Vagus Nerve

The enteric nervous system plays a profound part in the regulation of GI motility and secretion. Its receptors sense different chemicals present in foodstuffs, changes in muscle tension, and various peptides released from endocrine cells and nerves present in the gut. Approximately 75% of vagal fibers are afferent, and much of this information is relayed to vagal nuclei in the brain. In some cases this input causes an efferent signal also relayed by vagal nerves that results in a change in gut function—a so-called vagovagal reflex.

Most afferent vagal fibers pass through the nodose ganglion and terminate in the **nucleus tractus solitarius** (NTS) of the hindbrain. The hindbrain is able to regulate food intake in response to peripheral signals if input from higher centers is surgically eliminated.

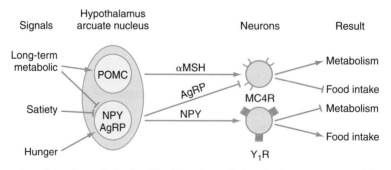

FIGURE 13-1 ■ Integration of signals regulating food intake and metabolism by the components of the arcuate nucleus of the hypothalamus. AgRP, agouti-related peptide; MC4R, melanocortin receptor; αMSH, α-melanocyte-stimulating hormone; NPY, neuropeptide Y; POMC, pro-opiomelanocortin.

Several peptides that stimulate satiety and decrease feeding are known to activate receptors present on **vagal afferents.** In addition, the vagus nerve relays signals initiated by distention of the stomach. Vagal signaling to the NTS is integrated with information received by the hypothalamus to produce the appropriate responses in feeding behavior and metabolism. Experiments in which vagal afferent activity was blocked either chemically or surgically demonstrated the importance of this pathway in the overall regulation of food intake. In these studies, the inhibition of sham feeding by nutrient infusion was prevented; the amount of material in the stomach no longer influenced meal size; and the effects of satiety hormones were eliminated.

THE ENDOCRINE SYSTEM

The endocrine system is concerned primarily with the long-term regulation of food intake and the maintenance of body weight. Normally, body weight is maintained within a relatively constant range over long periods of time despite changes in physical activity, metabolic demand, and caloric intake. For example, after an illness, humans increase food intake until lost weight is regained. Body weight then plateaus at or near the preillness level, and food intake returns to normal. The same phenomenon can be observed in animals that have been fasted or force-fed to cause weight loss or gain, respectively. In each case, when the animal is allowed to eat ad libitum, food intake either increases or decreases to bring body weight back to normal levels. Long-term appetite and body weight are now known to be regulated, at least in part, by hormones from the pancreas and adipose tissue. (Table 13-1 lists hormones believed to affect food intake in humans.)

Insulin

Insulin is produced by the beta cells of the endocrine pancreas and regulates glucose uptake, the storage of absorbed nutrients, and caloric or energy balance. Insulin can be transported across the blood-brain barrier and binds to receptors present in areas of the hypothalamus that control food intake. In patients with type 1 diabetes mellitus, the absence of adequate insulin is associated with increased food intake. In rodents, administration of insulin to the brain reduces food intake, whereas similar administration of insulin antibodies increases feeding behavior and weight gain. Additional evidence indicates that insulin potentiates satiety factors released from gut endocrine cells.

Leptin

Until the 1990s, fat was believed to do little but store calories and act as an insulator. In 1994 the discovery of **leptin,** an appetite-suppressing hormone secreted by fat cells, started a new era of research involving fat and the control of food intake. Leptin receptors have been identified on neurons present in both pathways in the arcuate nucleus of the hypothalamus. The pathway producing the appetite-stimulating peptides NPY and AgRP is inhibited by leptin, and the pathway producing POMC, which inhibits food intake, is stimulated by leptin. Leptin is also secreted from endocrine cells in the stomach in response to feeding and **cholecystokinin** (CCK). This is in contrast to the leptin found in fat cells that is released constitutively. Leptin receptors are also present on vagal afferent neurons. Disruption of leptin receptors in the hypothalamus produces only modest obesity compared with that of

TABLE 13-1			
Hormones Affecting Food Intake in Humans			
Hormone	**Source**	**Site of Action**	**Effect**
Insulin	Pancreatic beta cells	Hypothalamus	↓Appetite ↑Metabolism
Leptin	Fat cells Endocrine cells of the stomach	Hypothalamus ↓NPY, AgRP ↑POMC Vagal afferents	↓Appetite ↑Metabolism ↓Ghrelin release
CCK	I cells of the duodenum	Vagal afferents	↓Appetite ↓Gastric emptying
PYY	L cells of the ileum and colon	Hypothalamus ↓NPY, AgRP ↑POMC Stomach	↓Appetite ↑Metabolism ↓Gastric emptying
Ghrelin	Endocrine cells of the stomach Hypothalamus Large and small intestines	Hypothalamus ↑NPY, AgRP Vagal afferents	↑Appetite ↓Metabolism ↓Leptin release

AgRP, agouti-related peptide; CCK, cholecystokinin; NPY, neuropeptide Y; POMC, pro-opiomelanocortin; PYY, peptide YY.

total receptor knockout. This finding suggests that the effects of leptin on vagal afferent receptors are more important. Leptin has been demonstrated to increase the satiety response to CCK and may sensitize vagal afferent neurons to this gut hormone.

Thus leptin appears to be part of a negative feedback system for the regulation of food intake. As fat stores increase or during the response to a meal, more leptin is released, food intake is inhibited, and energy expenditure is increased. The discovery of leptin created great anticipation that it could be used to reduce food intake in obese persons, until investigators showed that most obese persons have high circulating levels of the hormone. Thus, although exogenous leptin reverses obesity in humans caused by its absence, leptin deficiency is not the usual reason for overeating and obesity.

THE GASTROINTESTINAL SYSTEM

Endocrine cells lining the GI tract are the source of several peptides known to regulate feeding behavior. Some peptides act on vagal afferents, thereby relaying information to the satiety center in the hindbrain. Others are transported through the blood-brain barrier and act directly on the hypothalamus. The information reaching these two centers is integrated into the overall satiety/hunger response.

Cholecystokinin

CCK was the first peptide shown to elicit satiety. In 1973 Smith, Young, and Gibbs showed that CCK injection caused rats to stop eating and begin grooming. This response occurred in animals with an open gastric fistula, which excluded gastric distention as a stimulus. As discussed in Chapter 1, CCK is released from I cells in the duodenal mucosa in response to fat and protein digestion products. CCK causes its inhibition of feeding by acting on vagal afferents because its effects are reduced by vagotomy or by chemical destruction of the vagal afferents with capsaicin. The effect of CCK also is inhibited by lesions of the NTS. CCK1 receptors are present on intestinal vagal afferents, a finding strongly supporting the idea that the short-term regulation of prandial satiety is largely the result of the release of CCK. The CCK1 receptors on vagal afferents transmit signals to the NTS, thus

decreasing the expression of melanin RNA and inhibiting the release of ghrelin and the expression of its receptor. One of the physiologic effects of CCK also is the inhibition of gastric emptying. This results in increased gastric distention and contributes to the satiety response. In humans, the infusion of CCK inhibits food intake and decreases feeding time, and the infusion of a CCK1 receptor antagonist produces the opposite effects. The arcuate nucleus of the hypothalamus and the NTS of the hindbrain are connected by reciprocally projecting neurons. Thus the long-term effects of centrally acting satiety hormones are potentiated by the short-term release of peripherally acting CCK.

Peptide YY

Peptide YY (PYY) is another candidate for a short-term satiety factor released from the gut. Like NPY, it is a member of the pancreatic polypeptide family and is produced as a 36–amino acid tyrosine containing peptide. PYY is released from enteroendocrine cells (L cells) of the ileum and colon by fat digestion products and may act to inhibit gastric emptying and secretion at the end of a meal. Circulating PYY reaches the hypothalamus via semipermeable capillaries of the median eminence to bind Y2 receptors, thereby inhibiting NPY neurons and releasing inhibition of POMC neurons. In humans, intravenous infusion of PYY in amounts yielding blood levels similar to those following a meal reduces food intake in both lean and obese persons. Obese persons have lower endogenous serum levels of PYY than do those in control subjects of normal weight. Unlike the case for leptin, persistent administration of PYY to obese subjects results in weight loss. Thus there is interest in PYY as a possible appetite suppressor. However, the overall significance of PYY both physiologically and clinically in the control of food intake has not been established.

Ghrelin

Ghrelin is a 28–amino acid peptide secreted primarily by endocrine cells in the oxyntic gland area of the stomach. Gastrectomy reduces plasma ghrelin levels by 65%, a finding indicating significant contributions from extragastric sites. These include the hypothalamus, small and large intestines, pancreas, and the kidney. Ghrelin binds to the growth hormone secretagogue receptor, stimulates the release of growth hormone from the pituitary, and increases the appetite, gastric motility, secretion of gastric acid, adipogenesis, and insulin secretion. Plasma levels of ghrelin increase during fasting, peak just before food intake begins or when the subject is expecting a meal, and fall within an hour of the start of feeding. Neither protein intake nor gastric distention associated with the intake of a meal inhibits ghrelin release. However, oral or intravenous glucose and a high-fat meal reduced plasma levels of ghrelin. In the hypothalamus, ghrelin stimulates neurons of the arcuate nucleus that express NPY. It also exerts actions directly on vagal afferents and on the dorsal vagal complex.

Plasma ghrelin levels correlate with a patient's nutritional status. Levels are high in lean people, and intravenous ghrelin increases food intake in persons of normal weight. Ghrelin plasma levels are low in obese persons and increase only after weight loss, a finding suggesting that increased circulating levels of the hormone are not responsible for overeating. Following bypass surgery for obesity, plasma ghrelin decreases further from already low levels, a response accompanied by decreased hunger. Patients with anorexia nervosa have high plasma levels, which return to normal after weight gain. Additional evidence from animal experiments indicates that ghrelin inhibits the release of leptin and that leptin has a negative influence on ghrelin release. A genetic deletion in mice that causes a defect in the mechanisms leading to satiety results in hyperphagia and abnormally high levels of plasma ghrelin. Taken together, these data indicate that ghrelin initiates the feeding response.

Additional Peptides

Other peptides from the GI tract have been shown to inhibit food intake and may have anorectic functions. Current research is in progress involving glucagon-like peptide 1 (GLP-1), oxyntomodulin (OXM), and pancreatic polypeptide (PP). In addition to inhibiting food intake, GLP-1 stimulates insulin release and inhibits gastric emptying. OXM, like GLP-1, is a product of the preproglucagon gene and has potent inhibitory effects on food intake in rodents. Its effects, however, are exerted on the arcuate nucleus, whereas those of GLP-1 are confined to the brainstem. PP reduces food intake in mice when it is administered peripherally, but central administration produces the opposite effect. In humans, PP inhibits the intake of food. Additional experiments are necessary to elucidate whether any of these peptides has a significant physiologic role in the regulation of caloric intake.

CLINICAL APPLICATIONS

Figure 13-2 presents the most likely approximation of current knowledge regarding the regulation of food intake. The agents shown, in addition to several others and/or their receptors, are candidates for the development of drugs to treat obesity. Leptin is effective in treating the rare cases of leptin deficiency, but resistance to the drug in the more common forms of obesity limits its usefulness. Two drugs are currently licensed to cause loss of weight. One of these inhibits pancreatic lipase and results in maldigestion and malabsorption of fat. The resulting steatorrhea is an unpleasant side effect, and the effectiveness of the drug is limited. The other acts centrally to prevent the reuptake of serotonin and norepinephrine. It also may have adverse side effects, although it does reduce appetite.

With greater frequency, obese patients with related health problems are turning to surgery as a means to lose weight. Weight reduction, or bariatric, surgery has proved to be a successful and permanent solution for many persons. The first procedures put into general practice were designed to decrease the absorption of ingested food by bypassing most of the absorptive surface of the small bowel. In the most popular of these procedures, called jejunoileal bypass, the intestine was transected near the duodenal-jejunal border, the jejunal end was closed, and the duodenal end was anastomosed to the distal ileum. The problems

Continued

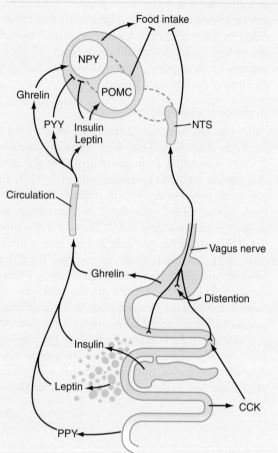

caused by malabsorption, however, made this procedure undesirable.

Currently, gastric bypass is the most commonly performed procedure. A small gastric pouch is created to receive esophageal content. It in turn is connected directly to the small intestine, so that the storage function of the stomach is eliminated, thus reducing food intake. Weight loss of 65% to 80% of excess body mass is typical of most patients. Medically more significant is a dramatic reduction in comorbidities. These include a correction in hyperlipidemia, decreased hypertension, improvement in obstructive sleep apnea, and a reduction in gastroesophageal reflux disease in almost all patients. Of major interest is a currently unexplained reversal of type 2 diabetes in up to 90% of patients that usually leads to normal levels of blood glucose without medication, sometimes within days following surgery. There was an 89% reduction in mortality over 5 years following surgery in a large clinical trial when compared with a nonoperated group of obese subjects.

FIGURE 13-2 ■ Summary of mechanisms involved in the regulation of food intake. CCK, cholecystokinin; NPY, neuropeptide Y; NTS, nucleus tractus solitarius; POMC, proopiomelanocortin; PYY, peptide YY.

SUMMARY

1. Obesity has become the number one health problem in the United States.
2. Our knowledge of the regulation of food intake is incomplete but has increased rapidly since 2000.
3. Food intake is regulated by the nervous, endocrine, and GI systems.
4. Satiety and hunger signals are integrated in centers in the arcuate nucleus of the hypothalamus and in the nucleus tractus solitarius of the hindbrain to regulate food intake and metabolism.
5. Long-term regulation is provided by the endocrine system in the form of insulin released from the pancreas and leptin released from fat cells. Both these hormones inhibit the appetite and thereby limit food intake.
6. GI peptides such as PYY, CCK, and ghrelin are short-term regulators of food intake. PYY acts on the arcuate nucleus to suppress the appetite,

whereas ghrelin acts on it to increase food intake. CCK and gastric distention activate vagal afferent fibers to the hindbrain to inhibit food intake and decrease the duration of a meal.

KEY WORDS AND CONCEPTS

Arcuate nucleus

Melanocortin

Neuropeptide Y

Nucleus tractus solitarius

Vagal afferents

Insulin

Leptin

Cholecystokinin

Peptide YY

Ghrelin

SUGGESTED READINGS

Badman MK, Flier JS: The gut and energy balance: visceral allies in the obesity wars, *Science* 307:1909–1914, 2005.

Blackman S: The enormity of obesity, *Scientist May* 24:20–24, 2004.

Chao C, Hellmich MR: Gastrointestinal peptides: gastrin, cholecystokinin, somatostatin, and ghrelin. In Johnson LR, editor: ed 5, *Physiology of the Gastrointestinal Tract*, vol 1, San Diego, 2012, Elsevier.

De Lartigue G, Raybould HE: The gastrointestinal tract and control of food intake. In Johnson LR, editor: ed 5, *Physiology of the Gastrointestinal Tract*, vol 2, San Diego, 2012, Elsevier.

Konturek SJ, Konturek JW, Pawlik T, Brzozowski T: Brain-gut axis and its role in the control of food intake, *J Physiol Pharmacol* 55:137–154, 2004.

Rindi G, Torsello A, Locatelli V, Solcia E: Ghrelin expression and actions: a novel peptide from an old cell type of the diffuse endocrine system, *Exp Biol Med* 229:1007–1016, 2004.

Stephens P: The endocrinology of pediatric obesity, *Endocr News* October:24-27, 2004.

REVIEW EXAMINATION

Multiple Choice

Select the best answer:

1. If a peptide belonging to the gastrin/cholecystokinin (CCK) family and having a sulfated tyrosyl residue in the seventh position from the C-terminus is desulfated, the most likely consequence for activity of the peptide will be
   a. a pattern of activity identical to that of gastrin.
   b. no change in pattern of activity.
   c. increased ability to stimulate gallbladder contraction.
   d. decreased ability to stimulate gastric acid secretion.
   e. a pattern of activity identical to that of CCK.

2. Gastrointestinal (GI) hormones
   a. stimulate their target cells from the luminal side of the gut.
   b. are for the most part inactivated as they pass through the liver.
   c. are released from discrete glands within the mucosa of the GI tract.
   d. pass through the liver and heart before reaching their targets.
   e. are bound to plasma proteins in the blood.

3. Cholecystokinin
   a. stimulates gastric emptying.
   b. is released by vagal stimulation.
   c. is released by protein and fat in the proximal small bowel.
   d. is released by distention when food enters the small bowel.
   e. is an important stimulator of gastric acid secretion.

4. Which of the following is *not* true about gastrinoma (Zollinger-Ellison syndrome)?
   a. Patients usually present with gastric ulcer.
   b. Patients develop diarrhea.
   c. Patients often have fat in their stools.
   d. Symptoms disappear after total gastrectomy.
   e. Following secretin injection, the levels of gastrin in the serum increase.

5. Stimulation of an intrinsic nerve in the intestine causes contraction of an intestinal muscle cell through the release of which neurotransmitter?
   a. Acetylcholine (ACh)
   b. Nitric oxide (NO)
   c. Norepinephrine
   d. Somatostatin
   e. Vasoactive intestinal peptide (VIP)

6. A nerve ending that releases NO onto a smooth muscle cell of the jejunum is injected with a dye that spreads throughout the nerve. The nerve cell body labeled by the dye most likely will be located in the
   a. brain.
   b. celiac ganglion.
   c. myenteric plexus.
   d. sacral region of the spinal cord.
   e. thoracic region of the spinal cord.

7. A muscle cell that has no striations and a ratio of thin to thick filaments of 15:1 most likely would be found in which region of the gastrointestinal tract?
   a. External anal sphincter
   b. Lower esophageal sphincter (LES)
   c. Pharynx
   d. Tongue
   e. Upper esophageal sphincter (UES)

8. In the presence of drug X, application of ACh to a bundle of gastric muscle cells causes membrane action potentials, an increase followed by a decrease in intracellular free calcium, but no contractile response. Drug X most likely is inhibiting which step in the contraction-relaxation process?
   a. Activation of myosin light chain kinase
   b. Binding of ACh with membrane receptors
   c. Opening of membrane calcium channels
   d. Opening of sarcoplasmic reticulum calcium channels
   e. Spread of excitation among muscle cells

9. A lesion is made that results in loss of primary peristaltic contractions of the pharynx and esophagus, but secondary peristalsis of the lower esophagus occurs on distention of the esophageal body. The lesion most likely is in the
   a. cortical region of the brain.
   b. cricopharyngeal muscle.
   c. enteric nerves.
   d. nucleus ambiguus of the vagus.
   e. pharyngeal muscle.

10. A segment of esophagus is removed and placed in a tissue bath. The circular muscle in the segment contracts tonically and relaxes on stimulation of the nerves intrinsic to the segment. The segment is most likely from which region of the esophagus?
    a. Distal body of the esophagus
    b. LES
    c. Middle body of the esophagus
    d. Proximal body of the esophagus
    e. UES

11. A catheter that monitors pressure at its tip is inserted through the nose and passed an unknown distance. Between swallows it records a pressure that is subatmospheric and fluctuates during the respiratory cycle, decreasing during inspiration and increasing during expiration. In which region is the catheter tip most likely located?
    a. Esophageal body above the diaphragm
    b. Esophageal body below the diaphragm
    c. LES
    d. Orad region of the stomach
    e. UES

12. A patient experiences gastric "fullness" after eating only a small quantity of food. Manometry reveals normal peristalsis in both the upper and lower esophagus, but no receptive relaxation of the orad stomach. These findings are best explained by a defect in the
    a. nucleus ambiguus of the brainstem.
    b. dorsal motor nucleus of the brainstem.
    c. vagal nerves.
    d. enteric nerves.
    e. celiac ganglion.

13. Contractions of the orad stomach, proximal and distal antrum, pylorus, and proximal duodenum are monitored in a subject during the emptying of two meals that are identical except for their fat content. Compared with the low-fat meal, the meal high in fat would elicit
    a. a decrease in the force of pyloric contractions.
    b. an increase in the force of peristaltic antral contractions.
    c. an increase in the number of peristaltic antral contractions.
    d. an increase in the number of segmenting duodenal contractions.
    e. an increase in the number of tonic contractions of the orad stomach.

14. Slow waves are recorded from the orad stomach, proximal and distal antrum, and proximal duodenum in a fasted subject. Slow waves recorded during the burst phase of the migrating motor complex (MMC), compared with slow waves recorded during the relaxed phase, are characterized by
    a. a decrease in the apparent propagation velocity of antral slow waves.
    b. a decrease in the frequency of duodenal slow waves.

    c. an increase in the amplitude of antral slow waves.

    d. an increase in the frequency of antral slow waves.

    e. the occurrence of slow waves in the orad stomach.

15. Compared with the gastric motility response to a meal in an individual with intact vagus nerves, the response in an individual whose vagus nerves have been cut at a level just above the diaphragm would be characterized by
    a. decreased emptying rate of liquids.
    b. decreased emptying rate of solids.
    c. increased accommodation of the meal.
    d. increased mechanical reduction of food particle size.
    e. increased mixing of contents.

16. The rate of gastric emptying of a mixed meal of solid foods and liquids would be decreased by
    a. blocking activation of receptors in the duodenal mucosa.
    b. enhanced tonic contraction of the orad stomach.
    c. infusing an isotonic solution of sodium chloride into the duodenum.
    d. infusing an isotonic solution of sodium chloride into the stomach.
    e. infusing an isotonic solution of sodium oleate into the duodenum.

17. A patient experiences a rapid rate of transit of contents from the duodenum to the cecum. What characteristic would contractions recorded at various loci of the small intestine exhibit during this time?
    a. Frequency greater than that of the slow wave
    b. Low in force
    c. Mostly peristaltic
    d. Mostly segmenting
    e. Mostly tonic

18. Intravenous injection of a hormone initiates a phase of intense sequential contractions of the proximal duodenum that appears to migrate slowly toward the cecum. Which hormone was most likely injected?
    a. CCK
    b. Gastrin
    c. Motilin
    d. Secretin
    e. VIP

19. A region of the intestine contracts weakly on stimulation of its extrinsic nerves. Distention of the region elicits a peristaltic reflex, but with weak contractions. Slow wave activity is absent. Taken together, these findings suggest a disorder of the
    a. enteric nerves.
    b. parasympathetic nerves.
    c. release of motilin.
    d. smooth muscle cells.
    e. sympathetic nerves.

20. A normal subject's small intestinal contractions are recorded from three loci spaced 5 cm apart. Over a period of 2 hours, contractions occur at each site seemingly at random, with the interval between any two contractions being 5 seconds or a multiple of 5 seconds. Only rarely do contractions at the three loci seem to be in sequence. These data indicate that
    a. contractions are being recorded from the ileum.
    b. the subject is in a fasted state.
    c. every slow wave is being accompanied by a contraction.
    d. the contractions are causing rapid aboral transit of contents.
    e. the contractions are mostly of the segmenting type.

21. Intraluminal pressure is monitored from a region of the colon that exhibits a relatively constant resting pressure of about 20 mm Hg. When an adjacent region of the colon is distended, resting pressure falls to near 0 and then increases slowly back toward 20 mm Hg even though the distention persists. The region being monitored is most likely the
    a. ascending colon.
    b. external anal sphincter.
    c. ileocecal sphincter.

d. internal anal sphincter.

e. transverse colon.

22. Segmental contractions of the colon
    a. increase in frequency in response to increased circulating levels of epinephrine.
    b. occur more often than do peristaltic contractions of the colon.
    c. occur at a higher frequency in the sigmoid colon than in the rectum.
    d. occur at a frequency that is higher than that for slow waves in the same region.
    e. are accompanied by the loss of haustral markings.

23. Relaxation of the ileocecal sphincter will occur during each of the following *except*
    a. eating a meal.
    b. distention of the ileum.
    c. distention of the colon.
    d. injection of gastrin.
    e. injection of CCK.

24. In a patient in whom resting tone of the internal anal sphincter is normal, distention of the rectum induces normal relaxation of the internal anal sphincter, no change in tone of the external anal sphincter, and no sensation of the urge to defecate. These findings are consistent with the finding of damage to the
    a. enteric nerves.
    b. internal anal sphincter.
    c. vagus nerve.
    d. spinal cord.
    e. transverse colon.

25. The digestive action of saliva on starch results from
    a. lactoferrin.
    b. lingual lipase.
    c. ptyalin.
    d. kallikrein.
    e. bradykinin.

26. At high rates of secretion, compared with low rates, saliva would have a lower concentration of
    a. Na^+.
    b. water.

c. Cl^-.

d. HCO_3^-

27. All of the following are characteristic of saliva *except* that
    a. it has a high K^+ concentration.
    b. there is a large volume of secretion relative to the weight of the glands.
    c. both parasympathetic and sympathetic stimulation increase its flow.
    d. it is hypotonic.
    e. it is primarily regulated by hormones.

28. Salivary secretion is inhibited by
    a. smell.
    b. taste.
    c. nausea.
    d. pressure of food in the mouth.
    e. sleep.

29. Which of the following substances or combinations will produce the highest rate of acid secretion? (Each compound is given at its half maximal dose.)
    a. Histamine
    b. Gastrin
    c. Gastrin plus secretin
    d. ACh
    e. Histamine plus gastrin

30. Acid secretion during the cephalic response to a meal
    a. fails to occur when the antrum is acidified.
    b. is triggered by the entrance of food into the stomach.
    c. is prevented by vagotomy.
    d. is inhibited by insulin injection.
    e. is stimulated only by ACh acting on the parietal cells.

31. Following the administration of histamine to a fasting individual, all of the following will occur within the parietal cells *except*
    a. a decreased number of tubulovesicles.
    b. increased carbonic anhydrase activity.
    c. increased H^+,K^+-adenosine triphosphatase (ATPase) activity.
    d. an increased number of mitochondria.
    e. an increased area devoted to the intracellular canaliculus.

32. According to the two-component hypothesis for gastric acid secretion, the H^+ concentration in gastric secretion increases with the rate of secretion because
    a. the volume of the oxyntic component increases.
    b. the concentration of H^+ being secreted by the parietal cells increases.
    c. the volume of the nonoxyntic component decreases.
    d. the secretion of Na^+ is inhibited.
    e. the secretion becomes hypertonic.

33. Antral gastrin release is stimulated by all of the following *except*
    a. bombesin gastrin-releasing peptide (GRP).
    b. ACh.
    c. fat in the stomach.
    d. protein digestion products in the stomach.
    e. distention of the antrum.

34. The presence of acid (pH <3) in the duodenum
    a. inhibits gastrin release via somatostatin.
    b. increases pancreatic bicarbonate secretion.
    c. decreases bile production.
    d. increases gastric acid secretion.
    e. inhibits pancreatic enzyme secretion.

35. In someone with a total absence of gastric parietal cells, one would expect to find each of the following *except*
    a. decreased digestion of dietary protein.
    b. decreased absorption of vitamin B_{12}.
    c. little or no pepsin activity.
    d. increased growth of gut bacteria.
    e. lower than normal pancreatic bicarbonate secretion.

36. Administration of a drug that blocks the H^+,K^+-ATPase of the parietal cells of a secreting stomach
    a. will have no effect on the volume of secretion.
    b. will increase the concentration of H^+ in the secretion.
    c. will decrease the concentration of Na^+ in the secretion.
    d. will decrease the pH of the gastric venous blood.
    e. will decrease the potential difference across the stomach.

37. The interruption of vagal afferent fibers from the stomach would
    a. decrease the acid secretory response to sham feeding.
    b. decrease the release of gastrin by digested protein.
    c. decrease acid secretion in response to distention.
    d. decrease the release of somatostatin.
    e. increase acid secretion in response to histamine.

38. Between meals, when the stomach is empty of food,
    a. it contains a large volume of juice with pH approximately equal to 5.
    b. gastrin release is inhibited by a strongly acidic solution.
    c. it contains a small volume of gastric juice with a pH near neutral.
    d. bombesin acts on the parietal cells to inhibit secretion.
    e. it secretes large volumes of weakly acidic juice.

39. During the cephalic phase
    a. secretin stimulates pepsin secretion.
    b. CCK stimulates pancreatic enzyme secretion.
    c. ACh stimulates the G cell to release gastrin.
    d. bombesin stimulates parietal cell secretion.
    e. ACh stimulates pancreatic enzyme secretion.

40. In humans, maximal rates of pancreatic bicarbonate secretion in response to a meal result from
    a. the effects of small amounts of secretin being potentiated by ACh and CCK.
    b. large amounts of secretin released from the duodenal mucosa.
    c. VIP acting on the ductule cells.
    d. potentiation between CCK and ACh released from vagovagal reflexes.
    e. potentiation between small amounts of secretin and gastrin.

41. Vagal stimulation
    a. potentiates the effect of CCK on pancreatic acinar cells.
    b. directly stimulates pancreatic enzyme secretion.

c. releases CCK from the duodenal mucosa.

d. inhibits the effect of secretin on pancreatic ductule cells.

e. releases secretin from duodenal mucosa.

42. Pancreatic enzyme secretion
   a. contains enzymes for the digestion of fat and protein but not carbohydrate.
   b. is primarily stimulated by secretin.
   c. is stimulated by pancreatic polypeptide.
   d. originates from the ductule cells.
   e. occurs primarily during the intestinal phase of the secretory response.

43. Pancreatic bicarbonate
   a. is secreted primarily from acinar cells.
   b. is secreted in quantities approximately equal to those of gastric acid.
   c. is stimulated primarily during the gastric phase of digestion.
   d. secretion causes an increase in the pH of pancreatic venous blood.
   e. ion concentrations in pancreatic juice decrease with increasing rates of volume secretion.

44. Pancreatic enzymes
   a. are synthesized in response to a secretory stimulus.
   b. are stored in Golgi vesicles.
   c. are secreted in response to carbohydrate in the duodenum.
   d. are secreted in response to sham feeding.
   e. are involved in the breakdown of disaccharides.

45. A sample of bile taken from the gallbladder is compared with a sample of bile collected as it is being secreted from the liver. Compared with hepatic bile, the gallbladder bile will differ in that its
   a. bile salt concentration will be less.
   b. cholesterol–bile salt ratio will be greater.
   c. osmolality will be greater.
   d. phospholipid concentration will be less.
   e. potassium concentration will be greater.

46. Bile acid A has a greater solubility in intestinal fluid than does bile acid B. Compared with bile acid B, bile acid A is more likely to be

a. a secondary bile acid.

b. a trihydroxy rather than a dihydroxy bile acid.

c. absorbed passively in the jejunum.

d. unconjugated.

e. undissociated.

47. When the distal ileum is removed, there will be an increase in bile acid
   a. levels in hepatic venous blood.
   b. levels in portal venous blood.
   c. secretion by hepatocytes.
   d. storage in the gallbladder.
   e. synthesis by hepatocytes.

48. As the bile secreted by the hepatocytes flows through the hepatic ducts on the way to the gallbladder, there is an increase in bile
   a. bicarbonate concentration.
   b. bilirubin content.
   c. chloride concentration.
   d. H^+ concentration.
   e. osmolality.

49. The rate of absorption of free galactose in the small intestine, initially occurring at a submaximal rate, would be
   a. increased by adding an equal amount of glucose to the lumen.
   b. decreased by adding amino acids to the lumen.
   c. decreased by adding fructose to the lumen.
   d. increased by the addition of trehalose to the lumen.
   e. decreased by hypoxia in the enterocytes.

50. Which of the following enzymes is located in the brush border and plays a role in protein digestion?
   a. α-Dextrinase
   b. Carboxypeptidase A
   c. Pepsin
   d. Enterokinase
   e. Lactase

51. Colipase facilitates fat assimilation by
   a. digesting triglycerides.
   b. transporting fatty acids across cell membranes.
   c. preventing the inactivation of lipase by bile salts.

d. converting prolipase to lipase.

e. binding fatty acids and monoglycerides after they have been absorbed by the enterocytes.

52. Most medium-chain fatty acids do not appear in chylomicrons because
   a. they are not absorbed by enterocytes.
   b. they are transported by fatty acid–binding proteins.
   c. they do not bind to apoproteins.
   d. triglycerides containing them are not digested by pancreatic lipase.
   e. they are absorbed directly into the blood.

53. In the absence of enterokinase, one would also expect a decrease in the activity of
   a. pepsin.
   b. lipase.
   c. chymotrypsin.
   d. amylase.
   e. sucrase.

54. Amino acids
   a. are primarily absorbed in the distal gut.
   b. are, for the most part, absorbed by passive mechanisms.
   c. compete with glucose for Na^+ during their absorption.
   d. appear in the blood more rapidly when presented to the gut as small peptides rather than as free amino acids.
   e. are produced in the lumen primarily by the action of endopeptidases.

55. Each of the following acts as a good emulsifying agent *except*
   a. cholesterol.
   b. bile salts.
   c. fatty acids.
   d. lecithin.
   e. dietary protein.

56. Colipase
   a. digests the ester link in 2-monoglycerides.
   b. is a brush border enzyme.
   c. has no enzymatic activity.
   d. lowers the pH optimum of pancreatic lipase to match that of duodenal contents.
   e. displaces pancreatic lipase from the surface of emulsion droplets.

57. The reason that patients with a congenital absence of one of the amino acid carriers do not become deficient in that amino acid is that
   a. the amino acid is absorbed by passive diffusion.
   b. the amino acid can make use of other carriers.
   c. the amino acid is absorbed by facilitated diffusion.
   d. peptides containing the amino acid are absorbed by different carriers.
   e. the amino acid is an essential amino acid.

58. Within the enterocytes
   a. triglycerides are resynthesized in the smooth endoplasmic reticulum.
   b. chylomicrons are synthesized in the smooth endoplasmic reticulum.
   c. fatty acid–binding protein transports long-chain fatty acids to the Golgi apparatus.
   d. triglycerides are synthesized from medium- and short-chain fatty acids.
   e. the major triglyceride resynthesis pathway makes use of dietary glycerol.

59. Of the 8 to 10 L of H_2O entering the digestive tract per day,
   a. only 100 to 200 mL is excreted in the stool.
   b. most comes from the diet (includes liquids).
   c. most is absorbed in the large intestine.
   d. gastric secretions contribute twice the volume of those from the pancreas.
   e. most is absorbed against its own concentration gradient.

60. In the small intestine, Na^+ is absorbed by each of the following processes *except*
   a. diffusion.
   b. coupled to amino acid absorption.
   c. coupled to galactose absorption.
   d. coupled to the transport of H^+ in the opposite direction.
   e. coupled to the absorption of HCO_3^-.

61. In the distal portion of the ileum,
   a. most fatty acids are absorbed.
   b. Cl^- is absorbed in exchange for HCO_3^-.
   c. Na^+ absorption occurs primarily coupled to glucose and amino acids.
   d. intrinsic factor is secreted.
   e. K^+ is absorbed in exchange for Na^+.

62. In the small intestine each of the following is true regarding Cl^- absorption *except that*
    a. it occurs down its electrical gradient.
    b. it occurs in exchange for Na^+.
    c. it occurs in exchange for HCO_3^-.
    d. it will result in the absorption of water.
    e. it occurs along the entire length of the small bowel.

63. Osmotic diarrhea may be the result of each of the following *except*
    a. cholera.
    b. lactase deficiency.
    c. inactivation of pancreatic lipase.
    d. Zollinger-Ellison syndrome (gastrinoma).
    e. loss of mucosal surface area in the small intestine.

64. Secretion of Cl^- by the small intestine
    a. occurs in exchange for HCO_3^-.
    b. takes place primarily in the villous cells.
    c. is inhibited by ouabain.
    d. produces an osmotic diarrhea.
    e. depends on an ATPase in the brush border membrane.

Matching

    a. Gastrin
    b. CCK
    c. Somatostatin
    d. Secretin
    e. VIP
    f. Histamine

65. Inhibits gastrin release when antrum is acidified

66. Inhibits parietal cell secretion of acid when antrum is acidified

67. Stimulates growth of gastric mucosa

68. Released by gastrin and acts as a paracrine to stimulate acid secretion

69. Stimulates gallbladder contraction in response to fat in the duodenum

70. Stimulates intestinal secretion and relaxes smooth muscle

ANSWERS

1. A	17. C	33. C	49. E	65. C
2. D	18. C	34. B	50. D	66. C
3. C	19. D	35. A	51. C	67. A
4. A	20. E	36. D	52. E	68. F
5. A	21. D	37. C	53. C	69. B
6. C	22. B	38. B	54. D	70. E
7. B	23. C	39. E	55. A	
8. A	24. D	40. A	56. C	
9. D	25. C	41. B	57. D	
10. B	26. B	42. E	58. A	
11. A	27. E	43. B	59. A	
12. C	28. E	44. D	60. E	
13. D	29. E	45. E	61. B	
14. C	30. C	46. B	62. B	
15. B	31. D	47. E	63. A	
16. E	32. A	48. A	64. C	

INDEX

Page numbers followed by *f* indicate figures; *t*, tables; *b*, boxes.